FRCS Trauma and Orthopaedics Viva

T0201877

OXFORD HIGHER SPECIALTY TRAINING

FRCS Trauma and Orthopaedics Viva

SECOND EDITION

EDITED BY

Nev Davies FRCS (Tr&Orth)
Consultant in Trauma and Orthopaedics, The Royal Berkshire Hospital, Reading, UK

Will Jackson FRCS (Tr&Orth)
Consultant, Nuffield Department of Orthopaedics, Rheumatology and Musculoskeletal Sciences, Oxford
University, Oxford, UK

Andrew Price DPhil, FRCS (Tr&Orth)
Professor and Honorary Clinical Lecturer, Nuffield Department of Orthopaedics, Rheumatology and
Musculoskeletal Sciences, Oxford University, Oxford, UK

Jonathan Rees MBBS, FRCS (Eng), MD, FRCS (Tr&Orth)
Director—Botnar Research Centre, University of Oxford; NIHR Senior Investigator—President British Elbow
and Shoulder Society, Oxford, UK

Chris Lavy OBE, MD, MCh, FRCS
Professor and Honorary Consultant Orthopaedic Surgeon, Nuffield Department of Orthopaedics,
Rheumatology and Musculoskeletal Sciences, Oxford University, Oxford, UK

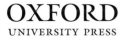

OXFORD
UNIVERSITY PRESS

OXFORD

UNIVERSITY PRESS

Great Clarendon Street, Oxford, OX2 6DP,
United Kingdom

Oxford University Press is a department of the University of Oxford.
It furthers the University's objective of excellence in research, scholarship,
and education by publishing worldwide. Oxford is a registered trade mark of
Oxford University Press in the UK and in certain other countries

First Edition published in 2012
Second Edition published in 2021
Impression: 1

Published in the United States of America by Oxford University Press
198 Madison Avenue, New York, NY 10016, United States of America

British Library Cataloguing in Publication Data
Data available

Library of Congress Control Number: 2021932653

ISBN 978–0–19–876624–7

DOI: 10.1093/med/9780198766247.001.0001

Printed and bound in the UK by
TJ Books Limited

Oxford University Press makes no representation, express or implied, that the
drug dosages in this book are correct. Readers must therefore always check
the product information and clinical procedures with the most up-to-date
published product information and data sheets provided by the manufacturers
and the most recent codes of conduct and safety regulations. The authors and
the publishers do not accept responsibility or legal liability for any errors in the
text or for the misuse or misapplication of material in this work. Except where
otherwise stated, drug dosages and recommendations are for the non-pregnant
adult who is not breast-feeding

Links to third party websites are provided by Oxford in good faith and
for information only. Oxford disclaims any responsibility for the materials
contained in any third party website referenced in this work.

Preface

In the surgical specialties we probably end up sitting more exams than any other profession. If you have purchased this book you are probably approaching the last serious exam that you will need to take. One of the problems is that it has now been several years since you sat a 'serious exam'. As such we are all at fault for building this next exam into something very big and very important, mainly because of the implications that failing has for both your professional and personal lives.

A number of your predecessors attended our clinical revision course in Oxford and one of the analogies we have always spoken about is being 'exam fit', the exam equivalent of the sporting 'match fitness'. As it is several years since you have taken an exam it is important to practise in exam situations and also to practise structuring answers to exam questions. If you do this for the first time in the real exam you will struggle. If it had been several years since you stopped playing a sport you would want and need a few second-team games before making your return to the first team—the same is true for this exam. So having revised over the last year or so and having passed your written exam you should have a good amount of core knowledge, but your 'exam training' should now be about seeing lots of clinical cases, practising your short-case technique, and importantly not forgetting to practise your viva technique. A wise professor once told us to revise in the way one is going to be examined, and this revision book is designed to help you to do this.

There are times when you might find it useful to read this book alone, but it has really been designed to be used in small groups. The philosophy of our course has always been that in the lead up to this particular exam you learn as much from watching and listening to your colleagues answer viva questions (in fact probably more!) as from answering them directly yourself. This book is therefore set out in a simple format with a starting clinical photograph, radiograph, or diagram and a set of questions followed by some suggested answers on the next page. Just as in a normal exam, the questions get more detailed as you progress further into the viva. The book allows you to work alone, with a colleague, or even with a team of colleagues who are taking the exam together.

During the viva exam it is quite easy to answer a seemingly difficult question (or even an easy question) in the wrong way and dig a very significant hole for yourself. It then becomes difficult to climb out of this hole; it affects your confidence and can have a detrimental effect on your performance. Remember, the examiners don't know you and you need to impress them with your safe, sensible, and knowledgeable approach to their questions. There are many different ways to start and respond to viva questions, and by watching and listening to a number of your colleagues answering these questions you will observe and learn that some methods are certainly safer than others. This book does not aim to tell you which methods to use, but working in groups allows further self-learning with regard to how you can plan to answer sensibly and safely, which is what your examiners are really looking for.

We hope you benefit from using this book; you are reminded that it is not a comprehensive knowledge text but an aid and approach to answering questions similar to the ones that you will encounter shortly in your exam. A final tip that we give to all candidates on our course is that when you are faced with that very very difficult clinical photograph or X-ray and you really have little idea of the very rare diagnosis before you, just 'say what you see'; this again reminds you that periods of silence in the exam do not score well but talking sensibly about what is in front of you will help you perform. We wish you the very best for your forthcoming exams and remind you that hard work now really does pay dividends for your future orthopaedic surgical career.

Nev Davies
Will Jackson
Andrew Price
Jonathan Rees
Chris Lavy

Acknowledgements

The editors and Oxford University Press would like to thank Paul Marks and FNS Publishing for the first publication of this book and their support. They would also like to thank Rachel Hubbard for her contribution to the first publication.

Contents

Contributors to the Second Edition

Taher Abdelrahman MBChB, MRCS, MSc, FRCS (Tr&Orth)
Sports Medicine Fellow, Fowler Kennedy, University of Western Ontario, London, Ontario;
Arthroplasty Fellow, University of Calgary, Calgary, Alberta; Arthroplasty Fellow, University of
British Columbia, Vancouver, Canada

Abtin Alvand BSc (Hons), MBBS, PhD, FRCS (Tr&Orth)
Consultant Knee Surgeon, Nuffield Orthopaedic Centre; Honorary Senior Clinical Lecturer in
Orthopaedic Surgery, University of Oxford, Oxford, UK

Kawaljit Dhaliwal MBBS, BSc, MRCS
Specialist Registrar in Trauma & Orthopaedics, KSS Deanery, UK

Amr Elkhouly FRCS, MCh, MBBCh
Consultant in Trauma & Orthopaedics, Royal Berkshire Hospital, Reading, UK

Paul Haggis MBBS, BSc (Hons), FRCS (Tr&Orth)
Locum Consultant Trauma & Orthopaedic Surgeon specializing in hip preservation, replacement,
and revision surgery, The Royal Cornwall Hospitals NHS Trust, Truro, UK
(Reviewer)

Luke D Jones DPhil (Oxon), FRCS (Tr&Orth)
Consultant in Trauma & Orthopaedics, Chelsea & Westminster Hospital, London, UK

Rebecca Mills BMBCh MA (Oxon), MRCS
Specialist Registrar in Trauma & Orthopaedics, KSS Deanery, UK

Paul Monk DPhil, FRCS (Tr&Orth)
Associate Professor, University of Auckland, Auckland, New Zealand; Honorary Lecturer in
Orthopaedics, and University of Oxford, Oxford, UK

Noel Peter BMedSci (Hons), BMBS, DipSportsMed, FRCS
Major Trauma Lead Honorary Senior Lecturer, NDS, University of Oxford; Consultant in Trauma
and Upper Limb Surgery, Cheltenham & Gloucester NHS Foundation Trust, UK

Daniel J Rolton FRCS (Tr&Orth)
Consultant Spine Surgeon, Royal Berkshire Hospital, Reading, UK

Huw Williams MBBS, BSc, MSc (Oxon), FRCS (Tr&Orth)
Upper Limb Fellow, Department of Orthopaedic Surgery & Musculoskeletal Medicine, University of
Otago, Christchurch, New Zealand

Contributors to the First Edition

Rachel Buckingham MB ChB, FRCS (Tr&Orth)
Orthopaedic Consultant, Nuffield Orthopaedic Centre, Oxford, UK

Peter Burge FRCS
Consultant Hand Surgeon, Nuffield Orthopaedic Centre, Oxford, UK

Jon Campion MBBS, BMedSci, FRCS
Consultant Orthopaedic Surgeon, Northampton General Hospital, Northampton, UK

Ramesh Chennagiri MS (Orth), FRCS (Orth), Dip Hand Surg (Br)
Consultant in Trauma & Orthopaedics, Wycombe Hospital, High Wycombe, UK

Paul Cooke MB ChM, FRCS
Consultant Orthopaedic Surgeon, Nuffield Orthopaedic Centre, Oxford, UK

Nev Davies BSc, FRCS (Tr&Orth)
Consultant Trauma & Orthopaedic Surgeon, The Royal Berkshire Hospital, Reading, UK

Mark Deakin MBBS, MSc, FRCS (Tr&Orth)
Consultant Trauma & Orthopaedic Surgeon, The John Radcliffe Hospital, Oxford, UK

Ad Gandhe BSc, MBBS, FRCS (Tr&Orth), DIP Graphics Design
Consultant Trauma & Orthopaedic Surgeon, Portsmouth Hospitals University NHS Trust, UK

Max Gibbons MA, FRCS
Consultant Orthopaedic Surgeon, Nuffield Orthopaedic Centre, Oxford, UK

Richie Gill BEng, DPhil
University Lecturer in Orthopaedic Engineering & Group Head of the OOEC, Botnar Research Centre, Nuffield Orthopaedic Centre, Oxford, UK

Siôn Glynn-Jones MA, DPhil, FRCS (Orth)
Professor of Orthopaedic Surgery, Nuffield Orthopaedic Centre/NDORMS, Oxford, UK

Roger Gundle MA, DPhil, FRCS (Orth)
Consultant Orthopaedic Surgeon, Nuffield Orthopaedic Centre, Oxford, UK

Steve Gwilym DPhil, MBBS, BSc, FRCS (Tr&Orth)
Associate Professor in Orthopaedics, University of Oxford; Consultant Trauma and Orthopaedic Surgeon, Oxford, UK

William Jackson FRCS (Tr&Orth)
Consultant Orthopaedic Surgeon, Nuffield Orthopaedic Centre, Oxford, UK

Chris Lavy OBE, MD, MCh, FRCS
Hon Consultant Orthopaedic Surgeon, Nuffield Orthopaedic Centre/NDORMS, Oxford, UK

Paul Marks BA, LLM, MD, FRCS
Consultant Spine/Neurosurgeon, Leeds General Infirmary, Leeds, UK

Rebecca Mills BMBCh, MA (Oxon), MRCS
Specialist Registrar in Trauma & Orthopaedics, KSS Deanery, UK

David Noyes FRCS (Tr&Orth)
Orthopaedic Trauma Consultant, The John Radcliffe Hospital, Oxford, UK

Andrew Price MA, DPhil, FRCS (Orth)
Professor of Orthopaedic Surgery and Consultant Orthopaedic Surgeon, Nuffield Orthopaedic
Centre/NDORMS, Oxford, UK

Jonathan Rees MBBS, FRCS (Eng), MD, FRCS (Tr&Orth)
Director—Botnar Research Centre, University of Oxford; NIHR Senior Investigator—President
British Elbow and Shoulder Society, Oxford, UK

Jeremy Reynolds FRCS (Tr&Orth), MB ChB, BSc (Hons)
Consultant Orthopaedic Surgeon, Nuffield Orthopaedic Centre, Oxford, UK

Aman Sharma MBBS, MRCSEd, MPhil (Cantab), MRCS
Spinal Research Fellow, Nuffield Orthopaedic Centre, Oxford, UK

Bob Sharp BMBCh, MA, FRCS (Tr&Orth)
Consultant Orthopaedic Surgeon, Nuffield Orthopaedic Centre, Oxford, UK

Tim Theologis MSc, PhD, FRCS
Consultant Orthopaedic Surgeon, Nuffield Orthopaedic Centre, Oxford, UK

Dionysios Trigkilidas BSc (Hons), MBBS, MRCS
Registrar in Trauma & Orthopaedics, Watford General Hospital, Watford, UK

Andrew Wainwright FRCS (Tr&Orth)
Consultant Orthopaedic Surgeon, Nuffield Orthopaedic Centre, Oxford, UK

Nick Ward MbChB, FRCS (Tr&Orth)
Consultant Trauma & Orthopaedic Surgeon, Frimley Park Hospital, Frimley, UK

Part 1   **Hands and Paediatric Orthopaedics**

Chapter 1 **Hands**

Viva 1

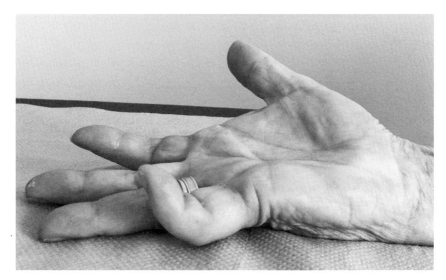

Figure 1.1 Clinical image of a right hand.

What is the likely diagnosis?

What is the epidemiology and risk factors for this condition?

What are the two main components seen in the histology of mature tissue from this condition?

Are there any ectopic manifestations?

What are the management options?

What are the risks of surgical treatment?

What is the likely diagnosis?

The clinical photograph shows a flexion contracture of the right little finger proximal interphalangeal (PIP) joint, suggestive of Dupuytren's disease.

What is the epidemiology and risk factors for this condition?

Dupuytren's disease is an autosomal dominant condition with variable penetrance. It is more common with age (fifth to seventh decade) in the male sex (7:1), and in northern European descendants. Associated risk factors include: positive family history, liver disease, high alcohol intake, diabetes mellitus, and epilepsy.

What are the two main components seen in the histology of mature tissue from this condition?

Histological appearance is the presence of myofibroblast cells and thick collagen fibres (type 3).

Are there any ectopic manifestations?

Ectopic manifestations include: Ledderhose disease (plantar fascia), Peyronie's disease (penis), and Garrod's knuckle pads on dorsum PIP joints. These manifestations may be associated with severe or aggressive Dupuytren's disease.

What are the management options?

The management options are non-operative measures and operative procedures.

Non-operative options include observation (and possibly splintage, especially at night).

Some authors have reported that steroid injections to early palmar nodules may reduce local tenderness. Although promising short-term results have been reported with collagenase injection, no long-term results are available.

Surgical options include:

- Percutaneous fasciotomy, especially for mild contractures affecting metacarpophalangeal (MCP) joint contractures or in patients medically unfit for general anaesthesia
- Segmental/palmar fasciectomy
- Regional fasciectomy (and Z-plasty closure or skin grafting)
- Dermo-fasciectomy and skin grafting
- PIP joint arthrodesis (for severe or recurrent disease)
- Occasionally, amputation of the digit (for severe or recurrent disease)

What are the risks of surgical treatment?

Specific surgical risks include:

- Delayed wound healing, infection
- Tendon, nerve, and vessel injury
- Haematoma and flap necrosis
- Temporary or permanent numbness
- Necrosis of the digit and amputation
- Incomplete correction
- Recurrence and re-operation
- Joint stiffness
- Reduced flexion/extension, especially at the PIP joint
- Pain, swelling, and tenderness; occasionally chronic regional pain syndrome

Viva 2

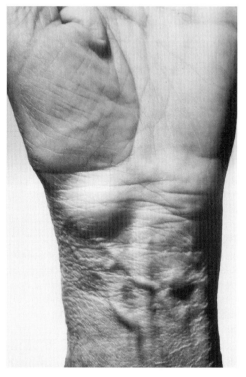

Figure 1.2 Clinical image of a wrist swelling.

Reproduced from C. Bulstrode et al., *Oxford Textbook of Trauma and Orthopaedics* second edition, 2011, figure 6.13.2, page 512, with permission from Oxford University Press.

What is the likely diagnosis of the cystic, soft-tissue lump shown in the photograph? From what structure does it commonly arise?

What clinical test, outpatient procedure, and simple imaging investigation can be performed to confirm the diagnosis?

Give a histological definition of this condition.

What are the other sites for these cystic swellings in the wrist and hand?

How would you manage this condition in a 26-year-old woman who works as a secretary and presents to you for the first time?

What is the risk of recurrence post-excision?

What is the likely diagnosis of the cystic, soft-tissue lump shown in the photograph? From what structure does it commonly arise?

The appearance of the lump at the wrist is suggestive of a ganglion cyst. Approximately two-thirds of such cysts originate in the radiocarpal joint. The remaining third arise from the scapho-trapezoid joint.

What clinical test, outpatient procedure, and simple imaging investigation can be performed to confirm the diagnosis?

Clinical test = compressible lump that trans-illuminates

Outpatient procedure = aspiration of the ganglion under local anaesthetic

Simple imaging investigation = ultrasound scan

Give a histological definition of this condition

A ganglion cyst is a fluid-filled cavity lined by compressed collagen and a few cells.

What are the other sites for these cystic swellings in the wrist and hand?

1. Ganglia in the hand are commonly seen over the dorsum of the wrist where they commonly arise from the scapho-lunate joint
2. Cysts arising from the distal interphalangeal (DIP) joint present as dorsal cysts and are called dorsal distal ganglia, mucoid, or mucous cysts and arise owing to osteoarthritis (OA) at the DIP joint
3. Smaller, firmer cysts may be found in relation to the flexor tendon sheath in the region of the A2 pulley. These are called palmar digital ganglia, flexor sheath ganglia, or pearl ganglia

Interosseous ganglia are uncommon, but when present are often in the lunate bone.

How would you manage this condition in a 26-year-old woman who works as a secretary and presents to you for the first time?

I would explain:

1. That a ganglion is a common benign cyst
2. That during the natural history of a ganglion it can often fluctuate in size periodically and may resolve spontaneously if simply observed
3. Treatment options and their potential risks include:
   - Simple observation (few if any risks)
   - Aspiration of the cyst (small risks of haematoma or infection, radial artery damage, and recurrence)
   - Surgical excision of the ganglion, open or arthroscopic (risks of anaesthesia and surgery include: nerve, vessel, tendon, and ligament injury, haematoma, infection, pain, swelling, tenderness, stiffness, and recurrence)

What is the risk of recurrence post-excision?

The risk of recurrence in some published series is similar for all three treatment options above, so observation is the safe course of action.

Viva 3

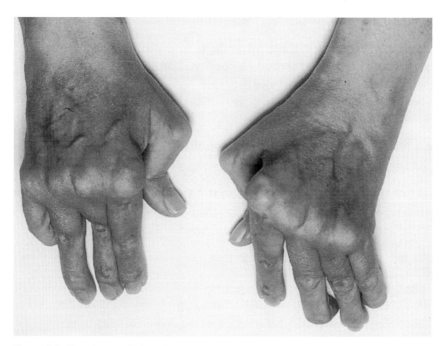

Figure 1.3 Clinical image of bilateral symmetrical hand deformity.

Describe the picture.

How would you grade this thumb condition radiologically?

Why does subluxation occur in this condition?

How could you explain the hyperextension deformity at the MCP joint?

What are the management options?

How would you treat this patient who has unremitting carpo-metacarpal (CMC) joint pain despite full non-operative treatment and who is fit for surgery?

What are the advantages and disadvantages and surgical risks with simple excision arthroplasty?

Describe the picture

This is a clinical photo of the dorsal aspect of the hands showing a symmetrical, deforming polyarthropathy consistent with rheumatoid arthritis. There are bilateral Z-shaped thumbs, swan-necking of the right middle finger, and marked ulnar deviation of all fingers at the MCP joints.

How would you grade this thumb condition radiologically?

I would use the Eaton and Littler system to stage this condition.

- Stage I—joint space widening, normal articular contours
- Stage II—slight narrowing of the CMC joint with sclerosis, up to one-third subluxation (on stress radiographs, thumbs resting on plate and pushing against each other): osteophytes < 2 mm
- Stage III—marked narrowing of CMC joint, more than one-third subluxation: osteophytes > 2 mm
- Stage IV—pan-trapezial arthritis [scapho-trapezio-trapezoidal (STT) joint involved]

Why does subluxation occur in this condition?

The palmar oblique ligament (also known as the 'beak' ligament) is a very strong ligament extending from the trapezium to the base of the first metacarpal. Degenerative attenuation and rupture of this ligament result in dorsal subluxation of the first metacarpal.

How could you explain the hyperextension deformity at the MCP joint?

Dorsal subluxation of the CMC joint causes metacarpal adduction, a thumb in the palm deformity, and reduction in thumb span. This leads to a secondary compensatory hyperextension at the MCP joint in an effort to increase the thumb span.

What are the management options?

Non-operative options include: oral analgesia; activity modification; use of splints; physiotherapy; and intra-articular steroid injection, which could be performed in the outpatient clinic or under fluoroscopic guidance.

Operative options include:

1. Excision of the trapezium offers satisfactory pain relief in most cases and preserves movement. Results are reliable. However, pinch grip may be weakened
2. The addition of a suspension procedure and tendon interposition [usually flexor carpi radialis (FCR)] has been shown to offer no extra benefit
3. First metacarpal-basal osteotomy may be considered, especially in earlier stages of the disease
4. Rarely, CMC arthrodesis is performed in young adult manual workers as this procedure offers a stable thumb with good pinch grip. However, the manoeuvrability of the thumb is affected
5. Implant arthroplasty has failed to offer good long-term results and early implant failure has made this procedure less popular

How would you treat this patient who has unremitting CMC joint pain despite full non-operative treatment and who is fit for surgery?

I would offer this patient excision of the trapezium and fusion of the MCP joint under general anaesthetic (GA)/regional block. I would perform the procedure as a day-case.

What are the advantages and disadvantages and surgical risks with simple excision arthroplasty?

Trapezium excision results in good pain relief and consequently improved function, but slight shortening of the thumb can cause reduced power of pinch. Risks specific to the procedure include: painful scar, infection, nerve damage (superficial branch of the radial nerve), blood vessel damage (radial artery), incomplete relief of symptoms (especially if adjacent joints are affected by osteoarthritis), a relatively slow recovery of function and attainment of maximal pain relief, and instability of the carpus.

Viva 4

A 20-year-old man presents 48 h after he was involved in a fight with another person, when he sustained a punching injury shown in the photograph below.

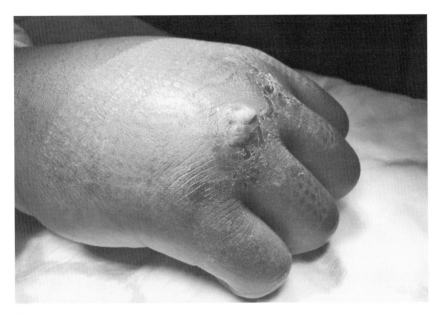

Figure 1.4 Clinical image of a ring finger injury.

What is the likely nature of this injury?

How would you assess this patient?

How would you treat this injury?

Which organism commonly causes infection with this type of injury?

Which antibiotics would you use to cover this organism?

What is the likely nature of this injury?

There is a 'fight-bite' puncture wound over the right ring finger MCP joint that may have been caused by a penetrating human tooth and may extend into the joint causing cartilage injury, bony fracture, and associated joint infection ± osteomyelitis.

How would you assess this patient?

I would take a full history including the circumstances of the injury, past medical history, and tetanus immunization status. I would look for systemic signs such as fever and tachycardia. On local examination, I would look for signs of cellulitis, tendon sheath infection, tendon rupture, and septic arthritis. I would request plain radiographs to exclude the presence of a foreign body and a fracture. I would also request baseline blood tests [full blood count (FBC), erythrocyte sedimentation rate (ESR), and C-reactive protein (CRP)].

How would you treat this injury?

My initial treatment would be to provide tetanus prophylaxis if indicated and apply sterile dressing to cover the wound. I would withhold antibiotics, if systemically well, until tissue samples are obtained. I would take the patient to theatre for urgent debridement under GA with a tourniquet around the arm. During surgery, I would obtain pus swab and tissue samples for histology and microbiological examination. I would extend the wound and look for tendon damage (re-create fist by flexing the MCP joint as the tendon can retract proximally). If the tendon is injured, I would not attempt primary repair. I would inspect the joint. I would then wash the wound with copious amounts of fluid. I would leave the wound open and apply a splint over non-adhesive dressing. I would commence broad-spectrum antibiotics, pending culture results and arrange for a further look after 48 h.

Which organism commonly causes infection with this type of injury?

Although *Eikenella corrodens* is peculiar to this injury, *Staphylococcus aureus* is the most common organism; other Gram-negative organisms may also be implicated.

Which antibiotics would you use to cover this organism?

I would prescribe broad-spectrum antibiotics according to local microbiological protocols such as co-amoxiclav, cephalosporin, and metronidazole.

Viva 5

A 24-year-old male cyclist has been knocked off his bicycle sustaining an isolated injury to his left wrist.

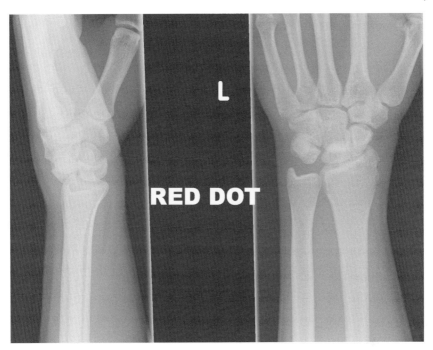

Figure 1.5 AP and lateral radiographs of a left wrist.

Describe the appearances of these radiographs.

How would you classify this injury?

What is the difference between a perilunate and a lunate dislocation?

How would you assess this patient's isolated injury?

Why does this injury need surgical repair?

How would you manage this injury initially and definitively?

How would you manage this injury in the chronic setting?

Describe the appearances of these radiographs

Postero-anterior (PA) and lateral radiographs of the left wrist showing a perilunate dislocation.
PA view shows:

1. Disruption of Gilula's smooth carpal lines that join the proximal joint surfaces of the proximal row of carpal bones at the radiocarpal joint and the distal joint surfaces of the proximal row of carpal bones and the proximal joint surfaces of the distal row of carpal bones (at the mid-carpal joint). The capitate appears to overlap the lunate
2. Hyperflexion of the scaphoid (scaphoid signet ring sign)
3. Abnormal triangular appearance of the lunate, but lunate located in the lunate fossa of the radius
4. Overlapping of the lunate and triquetrum [unable to visualize lunotriquetral (LT) joint]
5. No obvious fractures of radial styloid, scaphoid, capitate, triquetrum, hamate, or ulnar styloid

Lateral view shows:

1. Dorsal dislocation of the capitate head from its articulation with the lunate at the mid-carpal joint and dorsal translation of distal carpal row and metacarpals relative to the long axis of the radius

How would you classify this injury?

Perilunate injuries often follow a typical pattern as described by Mayfield. Assuming there are indeed no fractures, this is a 'lesser arc' ligament-rupturing perilunate dislocation. 'Greater arc' injuries also include one or more fractures, typically of the radial styloid, scaphoid, capitate, hamate, triquetrum (± ulnar styloid). A typical lesser arc perilunate injury follows the 'Mayfield sequence' of ligament failures in sequential defined stages:

Stage I: failure of the radiocarpal ligament
Stage II: failure of the scapholunate ligament
Stage III: failure of the LT ligament and dorsal mid-carpal dislocation
Stage IV: palmar dislocation of lunate at the radiocarpal joint (associated with median nerve compression)

Therefore this patient's injury is a Mayfield stage III lesser arc perilunate dislocation.

What is the difference between a perilunate and a lunate dislocation?

Perilunate = lunate stays in position and carpus dislocates. Lunate = lunate forced volar or dorsal while carpus remains aligned.

How would you assess this patient's isolated injury?

I would take a detailed history including handedness, occupation, mechanism of injury, co-morbidities, and time since last meal. I would examine carefully for abnormal wrist contour, pain, and swelling, and assess and document median nerve, sensory, and motor function.

Why does this injury need surgical repair?

Repair of the scapholunate ligament prevents a dorsal intercalated segment instability (DISI) deformity occurring, which leads to advanced arthritis of the radiocarpal and mid-carpal joints [scaphoid lunate advanced collapse (SLAC) wrist].

How would you manage this injury initially and definitively?

Initial management:

- Exclude another injury. Provide analgesia. Regular neurovascular observations
- Keep nil-by-mouth [± intravenous (IV) hydration if necessary]
- Splintage [e.g. padded plaster of Paris (POP) slap + loose bandage]
- High elevation (Bradford sling or Chinese finger traps)
- Explain severity of injury to patient
- Prepare and consent patient for urgent theatre
- Minimum initial intervention requires closed (± open) reduction of the dislocation using image intensifier control (± carpal tunnel decompression) + POP slab stabilization

Definitive intervention (± specialist hand surgery advice):

- Would include closed but anatomical restoration of carpal alignment using joystick k-wires (arthroscopically and image intensifier controlled) + buried k-wire stabilization of scapholunate, LT, and mid-carpal joints
- OR open dorsal anatomical carpal reduction, buried k-wire stabilization, and repair of scapholunate, LT, dorsal and palmar radiocarpal, ligaments
- Post-operatively: high elevation and careful neurovascular observation. Full POP for 6 weeks. Removal of wires at 8 weeks and mobilization
- Risks of post-traumatic carpal instability or stiffness ± OA

How would you manage this injury in the chronic setting?

I would assess the patient in a similar way. However, the surgical options would include a discussion with the patient about the merits of a proximal row carpectomy versus a total wrist fusion.

Viva 6

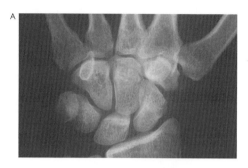

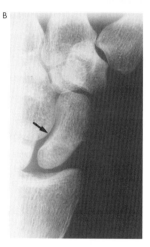

Figure 1.6 Left scaphoid radiographs.

Reproduced from C. Bulstrode et al., *Oxford Textbook of Trauma and Orthopaedics* second edition, 2011, figure 1.10.2, p. 75, with permission from Oxford University Press.

Describe these radiographs and explain the diagnosis.

What are the indications for internal fixation of scaphoid fractures?

Should acute non-displaced fractures be fixed?

What are the complications of this injury?

What is the blood supply to the scaphoid?

How would you plan the management of an established non-union of a scaphoid fracture?

Describe these radiographs and explain the diagnosis

The standard PA radiograph of the wrist does not show any obvious fractures; however, there is a subtle, non-displaced fracture of the scaphoid visible on the scaphoid view. This view is obtained by putting the hand and wrist in ulnar deviation, along with 15° of cephalad angulation of the X-ray tube. If there remains clinical suspicion despite normal radiography a computerized tomography (CT) should be considered.

What are the indications for internal fixation of scaphoid fractures?

Indications for internal fixation of a scaphoid fracture are:

1. If the displacement is > 1 mm
2. Or the scapholunate angle is > 60°
3. Lunocapitate angle > 15°
4. Intrascaphoid angle > 20° (dorsal humpback)
5. Proximal pole fractures, fractures associated with a perilunate dislocation
6. Delayed union

Should acute non-displaced fractures be fixed?

The overall rate of non-union scaphoid fractures treated in POP is 10%.

Not all acute non-displaced fractures need fixation, although there are some advantages. Studies have shown better early outcome scores, grip strength, and range of motion (ROM) with fixation, but no difference after 12–16 weeks. The rate of delayed union has been shown to be less with early fixation. Patients should be advised to avoid cigarette smoking to optimize their potential for bone healing.

What are the complications of this injury?

The two major complications related to this injury are avascular necrosis (AVN) of the proximal pole and non-union.

What is the blood supply to the scaphoid?

The proximal 80% of the scaphoid is supplied by retrograde blood flow from the dorsal carpal branch (radial artery), which enters the scaphoid in a non-articular ridge on the dorsal aspect surface. The distal 20% is supplied by the superficial palmar arch, which enters the distal tubercle.

How would you plan the management of an established non-union of a scaphoid fracture?

A CT scan will help to assess the amount of bridging trabeculae and the amount of union, identify a humpback deformity, any underlying wrist arthritis [scaphoid non-union advanced collapse (SNAC) wrist], and help to plan the size and shape of the bone graft required. If there is suspicion of AVN a magnetic resonance imaging (MRI) scan can be performed to assess blood supply.

If arthritic changes are not present on the radiographs, fixation with bone graft should be attempted in an effort to get the fracture to unite, decrease pain, and restore normal anatomy. Good results have been achieved in patients with AVN using vascularized distal radius bone graft based on the 1,2 intermetacarpal branch of the radial artery. If there is no AVN present autologous bone graft from the iliac crest can be used after fibrous tissue and sclerotic bone have been removed leaving vascular bone. A headless variable pitch screw can then be used for compression across the fracture to increase stability.

If arthritic changes are present and the patient is symptomatic, salvage procedures such as radial styloidectomy, proximal row carpectomy, scaphoid excision, and four-corner fusion and arthrodesis of the wrist should be considered.

Viva 7

This adolescent man comes to your clinic complaining of non-specific wrist pain with an MRI scan he has obtained privately.

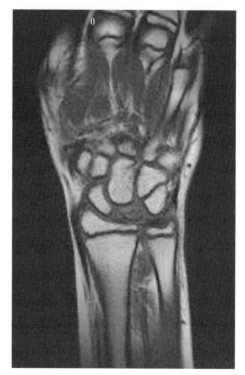

Figure 1.7 Coronal MRI image of a right wrist.

Describe what you see in the image.

What is the cause of this condition?

What is the staging system for this condition?

What else should you look for on the radiographs?

What are the management options?

Describe what you see in the image

This T1 MRI shows low signal density in the lunate, suggestive of Kienböck's disease.

What is the cause of this condition?

Kienböck's disease is AVN and subsequent disintegration of the lunate. Risk factors include: a history of trauma, ulnar negative variance (increases stress across the radiolunate), and vascular supply to the lunate.

What is the staging system for this condition?

The staging system for this condition is the Lichtmann classification, which recognizes four stages:

Stage I: normal radiographs, diagnosed on MRI/bone scan
Stage II: sclerosis of the lunate, no collapse
Stage IIIA: fragmentation and early collapse
Stage IIIB: IIIA + scapholunate dissociation and fixed rotation of the scaphoid
Stage IV: IIIB + degenerative changes in the wrist joint

What else should you look for on the radiographs?

I would look for negative ulnar variance on antero-posterior (AP) radiographs taken with the forearm in mid-prone position.

What are the management options?

The condition can be managed non-operatively with analgesia and splintage. Operative options include: joint levelling procedures (radius shortening), wrist denervation, partial or total wrist fusion, and proximal row carpectomy. Choice of treatment depends on the stage of the disease, degree of symptoms, and patient factors.

Viva 8

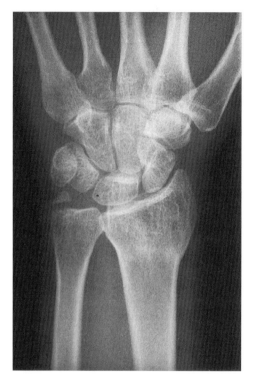

Figure 1.8 AP radiograph of a left wrist.

Reproduced from C. Bulstrode et al., *Oxford Textbook of Trauma and Orthopaedics* second edition, 2011, figure 6.4.9, p. 440, with permission from Oxford University Press.

Describe what you see on this radiograph of a 22-year-old with ulnar-sided wrist pain.

Which soft-tissue structure would you expect to be involved?

Can you simplify the anatomy of this complex structure?

How do you classify these injuries?

What are the management options for this condition?

What portals would you use in wrist arthroscopy and which structures do they put at risk?

Describe what you see on this radiograph of a 22-year-old with ulnar-sided wrist pain

This AP radiograph of the wrist shows ulnar positive variance. This appearance is typical of ulnar abutment syndrome.

Which soft-tissue structure would you expect to be involved?

Triangular fibrocartilage complex (TFCC) tears are frequently associated with this condition (Class 2).

Can you simplify the anatomy of this complex structure?

The TFCC is a pyramid-shaped fibrocartilagenous ligamentous structure found at the distal aspect of the ulna.

It comprises a fibrocartilagenous disc (a meniscus-like structure) and a sling of ligaments, and acts as a key stabilizer of the distal radioulnar (DRU) joint and the ulnocarpal joint.

The periphery of this structure is well vascularized with the remaining central portion being avascular.

How do you classify these injuries?

These injuries have been classified by Palmer into traumatic (Class 1) and degenerative (Class 2).

What are the management options for this condition?

Non-operative measures are splint, analgesia, and avoidance of aggravating activities. Operative options include: arthroscopic debridement, arthroscopic repair, ulnar shortening osteotomy, wafer resection of ulna, or Darrach procedure.

What portals would you use in wrist arthroscopy and which structures do they put at risk?

Portals are named in relation to the extensor compartment. I would perform a wrist arthroscopy under GA with a tourniquet and finger traps to the index and middle fingers connected to an overhead traction device. I would then identify the 3–4 portal by feeling for Lister's tubercle and going 1 cm distal to this, feeling for the soft spot and insufflating the joint with saline. I would then make a skin incision followed by blunt haemostat dissection. The 3–4 portal is established first and is the primary viewing portal. Extensor pollicis longus (EPL) and extensor digitorum communis (EDC) tendons are the structures at risk. I would then identify the 6R and 6U portals, which are used as primary adjuncts for visualization and instrumentation. They place the dorsal sensory branch of the ulnar nerve at risk.

Other commonly used portals include: the mid-carpal portals, Mid-Carpal-Radial (MCR), and Mid-Carpal-Ulnar (MCU). MCR is located 1 cm distal to the 3–4 portal along the axis of the radial border of the middle finger. Extensor carpi radialis brevis (ECRB) and EDC are at risk with this portal. MCU is located 1 cm distal to the 4–5 portal along the long axis of the ring finger metacarpal. EDC and extensor digiti minimi (EDM) tendons are at risk with this portal.

Viva 9

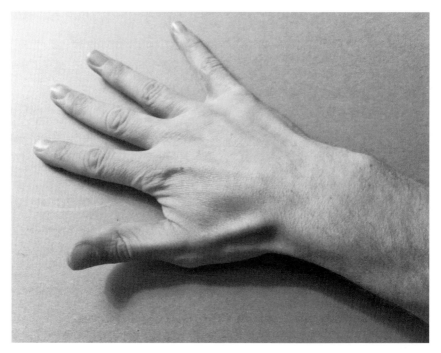

Figure 1.9 Clinical image of a right hand.

Tell me about the dorsal compartments at the wrist joint.

What is de Quervain's syndrome?

What are the clinical signs of de Quervain's syndrome?

What are the management options for de Quervain's syndrome?

What are the adverse effects of local steroid injection?

What are the pitfalls of surgery?

Tell me about the dorsal compartments at the wrist joint

There are six compartments in which the extensor tendons traverse the dorsum of the wrist:

1. APL, EPB (abductor pollicis longus, extensor pollicis brevis)
2. ECRL, ECRB (extensor carpi radialis longus, extensor carpi radialis brevis)
3. EPL (extensor pollicis longus)
4. EI, EDC (extensor indicis, extensor digitorum communis)
5. EDM (extensor digiti minimi)
6. ECU (extensor carpi ulnaris)

What is de Quervain's syndrome?

It is a painful condition affecting the first compartment tendons of the wrist joint. It is more common in females, especially post-partum.

What are the clinical signs of de Quervain's syndrome?

There is localized tenderness and/or swelling along the radial aspect of the wrist over APL/EPB. The Finkelstein test is considered positive if pain is elicited on holding the thumb and quickly ulnar-deviating the wrist. Pain may also be elicited on ulnar-deviating the wrist with fingers flexed over the thumb held in the palm.

What are the management options for de Quervain's syndrome?

Non-operative options are splintage, analgesia, and local steroid injection. If non-operative measures fail, I would proceed with surgical release under GA or regional anaesthetic and with an upper arm tourniquet. Release may be achieved through a longitudinal or transverse skin incision. I would perform this via longitudinal incision and then identify and protect the superficial branch of the radial nerve. Then I would divide the annular ligament ensuring all the compartments are decompressed. Finally, I would assess the floor of the compartment to look for any pathology.

What are the adverse effects of local steroid injection?

Adverse effects of local steroid injection are infection, skin atrophy and depigmentation, subcutaneous fat atrophy at the site of injection, injury to the superficial branch of the radial nerve (painful neuroma), and tendon rupture.

What are the pitfalls of surgery?

Failure to recognize anatomical variation (EPB may lie in a separate compartment) may lead to incomplete relief of symptoms. Injury to the sensory branch of the radial nerve could result in a painful neuroma.

Viva 10

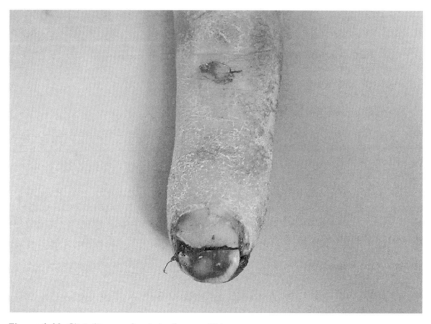

Figure 1.10 Clinical image of an index finger nail injury.

Reproduced from C. Bulstrode et al., *Oxford Textbook of Trauma and Orthopaedics* second edition, 2011, figure 14.7.1, p. 1675, with permission from Oxford University Press.

How would you manage this crush injury?

What would you explain to the patient?

How would you manage this crush injury?

I would take a relevant history, including: handedness, occupation, mechanism of injury, and co-morbidities. I would provide tetanus prophylaxis (if indicated) and antiseptic (betadine) dressing. I would obtain radiographs to exclude an underlying fracture.

As definitive management, I would explore and repair the nail bed under local anaesthesia (digital block) and digital tourniquet.

The salient steps of the procedure are:

1. Remove the nail plate carefully
2. Inspect the nail bed and wash thoroughly
3. Copious lavage of any underlying fracture
4. Reduce fracture if present and stabilize (axial k-wire; remove after 3–4 weeks) if necessary
5. Repair nail bed with a 6-0 absorbable suture (VICRYL Rapide)
6. Wash and replace nail plate. Figure-of-eight stitch (or equivalent) to hold the nail plate in place

What would you explain to the patient?

I would explain that the nail plate will fall off and be gradually replaced by a new one, which may initially appear disfigured. There is a risk of some long-term nail deformity (hook or split nail) and discomfort in the region of the nail bed and some distal interphalangeal joint stiffness.

Viva 11

This 26-year-old man presents to your clinic with a right thumb injury sustained while playing rugby.

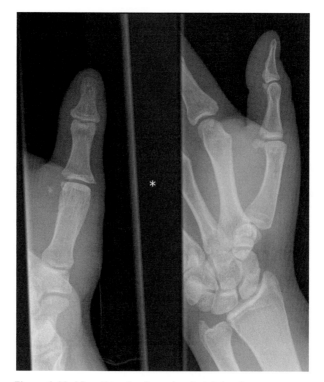

Figure 1.11 AP and lateral radiographs of a left thumb.

Describe the radiographs and explain the diagnosis.

Describe the anatomy and how you would examine it.

What is a Stener lesion?

What are the management options for an acute injury?

What are the management options for a chronic injury?

Describe the radiographs and explain the diagnosis

This is an AP radiograph showing a displaced avulsion fracture of the proximal phalanx on the ulnar aspect of the left thumb. This would indicate an injury to the ulnar collateral ligament (UCL) of the thumb MCP joint. These injuries occur when a valgus force in abduction is applied to the thumb, and can present acutely with trauma ('skier's thumb') or owing to chronic laxity ('gamekeeper's thumb').

Describe the anatomy and how you would examine it

The UCL is composed of a proper and accessory ligament. The proper collateral ligament resists valgus load with the thumb in flexion and the accessory resists valgus load in extension. These can be examined by stressing the joint in radial deviation in both neutral (accessory) and 30° of flexion (proper). The loss of an end point or more than 30° compared to the other side indicates a complete rupture.

The UCL originates from the medial condyle metacarpal and passes obliquely and volarly inserting into the volar third of the proximal phalanx and volar plate. The adductor aponeurosis is superficial to the UCL and inserts into the ulna border thumb extensor mechanism via the ulna sesamoid.

What is a Stener lesion?

It occurs in the presence of an UCL injury. The adductor pollicis aponeurosis becomes interposed between the ruptured UCL of the thumb and its site of insertion at the base of the proximal phalanx. This prevents the UCL healing.

What are the management options for an acute injury?

The management options include non-operative measures and operative treatment. Non-operative management involves immobilization in a thumb spica for 4–6 weeks and is indicated for partial tears with a definite end point on stressing, an undisplaced complete tear, or an undisplaced bony fragment. Surgical treatment involves repair of the ligament by sutures, suture anchors, or screw fixation. Surgery is indicated for displaced complete tears, displaced bony fragment, presence of a Stener lesion, and chronic injuries.

What are the management options for a chronic injury?

Chronic injuries require reconstruction of the ligament by using a dynamic tendon transfer (adductor pollicis), a free tendon graft (palmaris longus), or a static tendon transfer (EPB).

Viva 12

This 46-year-old man is referred to your clinic with pain over the hypothenar area of his hand.

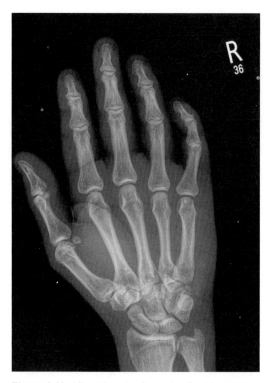

Figure 1.12 AP and lateral radiographs of a right wrist.

Describe the radiographic findings.

How would you manage this?

What is Guyon's canal?

What is ulnar tunnel syndrome?

What is the management?

Describe the radiographic findings

This is an AP radiograph showing a displaced hook of hamate fracture. This fracture is best identified on a carpal tunnel view. Plain radiography only picks up 40% of hamate fractures and a CT should be considered after a negative finding if clinically indicated.

How would you manage this?

I would take a full history and examine the patient. I would ask about hand dominance, occupation, and hobbies. Acute injuries can be immobilized for 6 weeks. Operative management includes excision of the hamate fracture or open reduction and internal fixation (ORIF). Better outcomes and ability to return to pre-injury activities have been found with excision of the fracture fragment compared with ORIF.

What is Guyon's canal?

Guyon's canal is a tunnel that is approximately 4 cm long, beginning at the transverse carpal ligament and ending at the aponeurotic arch of the hypothenar muscle. The canal is formed by:

Roof—volar carpal ligament
Floor—transverse carpal ligament
Ulnar border—pisiform and pisohamate ligament
Radial border—hook of hamate
Contents include: ulnar nerve and artery

What is ulnar tunnel syndrome?

Compression of the ulnar nerve in Guyon's canal. Within the canal, at the distal margin the ulna divides into a superficial sensory branch and a deep motor branch. Causes include: ganglia (from triquetrohamate joint), mass, hook of hamate fracture, ulnar artery aneurysm, or thrombosis. Compression can involve both motor and sensory symptoms (zone 1), motor symptoms only (zone 2), or sensory symptoms only (zone 3).

What is the management?

Managed options are non-operative measures and operative procedures. Conservative management involves restricting exacerbating exercises, splinting in neutral, and analgesia. Operative management involves surgical release.

Chapter 2 **Paediatric Orthopaedics**

Viva 13

This 2½-year-old girl is referred to your clinic with a limp.

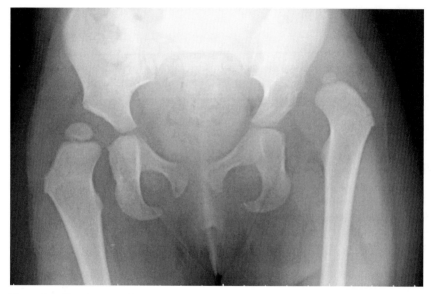

Figure 2.1 AP radiograph of a pelvis.

Describe the radiographic findings.

How would you proceed in your management from here?

What open operative approaches would you use to reduce this hip?

Describe the radiographic findings

This is an antero-posterior (AP) pelvic radiograph showing a dislocated left hip and dysplastic acetabulum. Shenton's line is broken and the femoral head lies lateral and superior to the inferomedial quadrant (made by the intersection of Perkin's and Hilgenreiner's lines).

How would you proceed in your management from here?

I would take a full history and examine the child. There may be risk factors for developmental dysplasia of the hip (DDH) including positive family history, female sex, and/or decreased intrauterine space (first born, breech, oligohydramnios).

More importantly I would be looking to see if there were any underlying neuromuscular conditions such as spina bifida, arthrogryposis, or cerebral palsy. Examination may reveal a Trendelenburg gait, leg length discrepancy, fixed flexion deformity, as well as reduced abduction of the left hip, which is the most consistent and reliable clinical sign of this condition.

I would organize an examination under anaesthesia (EUA) and arthrogram to delineate the anatomy of the acetabulum, soft tissues, and proximal femur. It would be unlikely that this hip would reduce closed. Indications for open reduction are failure of closed reduction or an unstable/incongruent reducible hip. The soft-tissue blocks to reduction that may need to be addressed include: adductor longus, iliopsoas, capsule, ligamentum teres, transverse acetabular ligament, pulvinar (fibro-fatty debris), inverted labrum, and limbus.

What open operative approaches would you use to reduce this hip?

I would use a modified anterior (iliofemoral or Smith-Peterson) approach to the hip. I would place my skin incision parallel and distal to the iliac crest, passing 2 cm distal to the anterior superior iliac spine (ASIS) and extending medially within the groin skin crease.

I would identify and protect the lateral cutaneous nerve of the thigh and then distally I would develop the internervous plane between the tensor fascia lata (superior gluteal nerve) and the sartorius (femoral nerve). Splitting the iliac crest apophysis, I would elevate the muscles *en masse* on both sides of the pelvis down to the sciatic notch and the superior border of the acetabulum. I would divide the straight head of the rectus femoris and then make a T-shaped capsular incision to enter the hip joint and clear the acetabulum of pulvinar and redundant ligamentum teres (not the labrum). Any inverted labrum will need to be everted and one or more radial cuts may be necessary to allow this. The inferior capsule may also require release, with care not to damage the blood supply to the femoral head. There is likely to be tightness of the iliopsoas and its tendon may need releasing in order to reduce the hip.

I would then assess the need for: (1) a shortening femoral osteotomy; and/or (2) pelvic osteotomy (e.g. Salter) to give more cover.

I would then perform a double-breasted capsular repair, close in layers, and apply a hip spica cast with the hip in approximately 30° of abduction and internal rotation. The spica would need changing at 6 weeks for a total of 3 months. Post-operatively, I would watch carefully for spica syndrome and organize a magnetic resonance imaging (MRI) scan to ensure the hip remains located.

The patient would require long-term follow-up to check that the hip develops normally.

Viva 14

This is a photograph of a 7-year-old girl sitting in a comfortable position. Her mother is concerned because she walks with her feet turned in.

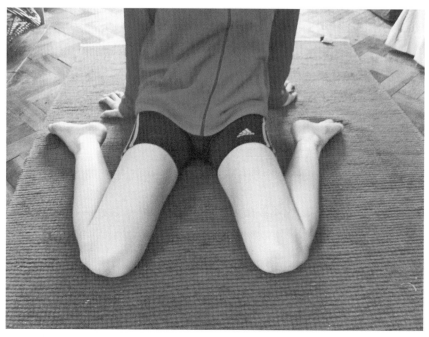

Figure 2.2 Clinical image of a 7-year-old girl sitting comfortably.
Photograph courtesy of Paul Thornton-Bott FRCS (Tr&Orth)

How would you proceed with your assessment?

You find on your examination that the child has extremely lax ligaments and increased internal rotation of both hips.

How do you grade ligamentous laxity in children?

The mother has asked about surgical treatment for this condition. What would you offer her?

How would you proceed with your assessment?

This clinical photograph shows a child sitting in the 'W' position.

Important questions in the history would include: enquiry about the pregnancy and birth, developmental milestones, family history, and any significant past medical history. I would ask the child and parents about current symptoms and concerns. The common causes of an in-toeing gait include: metatarsus adductus, internal tibial torsion, and persistent femoral anteversion.

In the examination it is important to rule out asymmetry in the lower legs or any neurological signs, which could indicate an underlying spinal abnormality or neurological problem.

I would examine the gait (with shoes on and barefoot), looking specifically at the foot progression angle (negative in this case: normal is −5° to +20°).

With the child lying prone I would assess the torsional profile, looking for:

- Metatarsus adductus: adducted forefoot, with a curved lateral foot border (rather than straight), normal hindfoot movement
- Tibial torsion: thigh–foot angle in prone position > 10° internal rotation (normal range 0–20° external rotation)
- Femoral anteversion: internal rotation > 70° (normal range 30–60°) and reduced external rotation < 20°

I would also examine the spine, lower limb neurology, and assess ligamentous laxity.

How do you grade ligamentous laxity in children?

I would use the Beighton scale, testing hyperextension in the upper limb and forward flexion of the trunk (a score of 5 or more out of 9 indicates hyperlaxity).

The mother has asked about surgical treatment for this condition. What would you offer her?

This child's in-toeing gait is most likely due to persistent femoral anteversion, which is a common cause in children older than 3 years.

I would reassure the mother that her daughter is physiologically normal and just at one end of the normal spectrum for children of her age. She may be interested to learn that the only effective treatment is to cut the femora, rotate, and then fix them, which is a major surgical procedure, with significant risks, for essentially a cosmetic problem.

I would also explain the natural history of the condition—that it tends to improve over the first decade but she may well be left in-toeing as an adult. As muscle balance improves into adulthood it rarely presents a functional problem.

Viva 15

This 13-year-old boy presented with pain in his right knee.

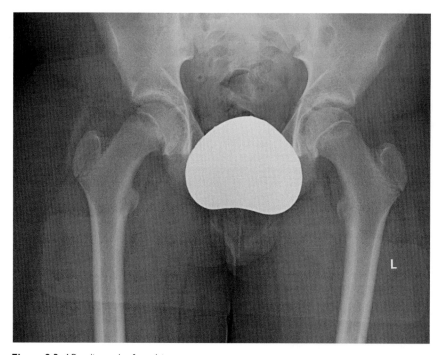

Figure 2.3 AP radiograph of a pelvis.

Describe the radiograph.

How do you classify this condition?

What is your management plan for the right hip?

What is your management plan for the left hip?

Describe the radiograph

This is an AP radiograph of the pelvis in a skeletally immature child. There is a mild slip of the right upper femoral epiphysis (SUFE) with a positive Trethowan's sign. This is shown by drawing Klein's line up the lateral border of the femoral neck and noting it does not intersect the epiphysis. Widening of the physis is also visible.

How do you classify this condition?

I would use Loder's classification, which divides SUFEs into stable and unstable based on the patient's ability to bear weight with or without crutches secondary to pain, and is useful for predicting the risk of avascular necrosis (AVN). SUFEs can also be classified into acute (symptoms < 3 weeks), chronic, or acute-on-chronic. The Southwick angle classification grades the degree of slip compared with the unaffected side into mild (< 30%), moderate (30–50%), or severe (> 50%) and is used to decide which can be pinned *in situ*.

What is your management plan for the right hip?

I would take a full history from the patient and parents and examine the child. I would particularly look for any associated endocrine disorders such as hypothyroidism or chronic renal failure in children under 10 or those with a weight below the 50th percentile.

Examination findings would reveal classically a hip that externally rotates and abducts with flexion.

My management plan would be to pin this slip *in situ* with a single cannulated screw, which has sufficient stability and a reduced risk of AVN compared with multiple screws. I would perform this under general anaesthetic (GA) on a fracture table, but would not use a forced reduction manoeuvre or traction, which might increase the risk of AVN. I would use a triangulation technique to define the appropriate location for the skin incision. The thread of the screw should be in the centre of the epiphysis passing through perpendicular to the physis (this avoids perforating the femoral head). As the slip is usually postero-medial, this technique usually requires an anterior femoral neck entry point. A minimum of three screw threads should pass into the epiphysis. The tip of the screw should be at least 5 mm from the subchondral bone on all views.

What is your management plan for the left hip?

Contralateral prophylactic screw fixation to prevent slip in the future remains a controversial topic. Options are to treat every case with contralateral fixation, versus pinning only those children thought to be at higher risk of contralateral slip or significant leg length discrepancy (less than 10 years old, underlying endocrinopathy, obese males).

Viva 16

This 8-month-old baby was brought to casualty with the below injury.

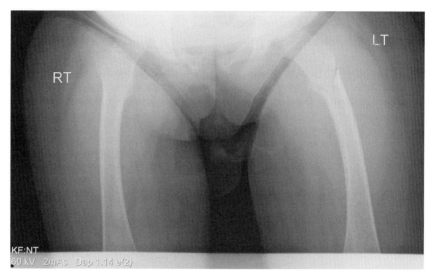

Figure 2.4 AP radiograph of proximal femurs.

What are your thoughts?

Tell me about non-accidental injury and what you would do if you suspected it.

How would you treat this fracture?

What are your thoughts?

This is a AP radiograph of a child's lower pelvis and femurs showing an oblique fracture at the left subtrochanteric level. I would like to take a detailed history from the parents or carer, as a femoral fracture in a non-ambulant child could be a non-accidental injury (NAI). You must pick this possibility up—it is reasonable for this to be a pass/fail type question.

Tell me about non-accidental injury and what you would do if you suspected it

NAI is an injury deliberately inflicted by a parent or a caregiver. It may be difficult to suspect a parent or carer of abuse but we have a duty of care as professionals to ensure care and protection of children.

Child abuse itself can take different forms (neglect, physical, sexual, psychological): most are in combination. It is the second most common cause of death in young children (after trauma). Risk factors include: first born, premature babies, children with disabilities, stepchildren, and family history of abuse.

First it is important to get the child into a safe environment and treat the traumatic injuries appropriately in the same way as for an accidental injury, according to Advanced Trauma Life Support (ATLS) guidelines and being mindful that there may be other more life-threatening injuries (subdural haematoma and 'shaken baby' syndrome). Having taken a detailed history from the parents and examined the child fully (with a chaperone), I would document my findings carefully in the notes and arrange a skeletal survey. Clues suggesting NAI in the clinical assessment include: a history that doesn't fit the injury, inconsistent explanations and delayed presentation, bruising patterns on the child, and retinal haemorrhages. I would inform the paediatricians of my concerns and make arrangements for the child to be admitted.

Radiographic clues for NAI include: metaphyseal bucket handle/corner fractures (virtually pathognomonic), rib fractures, and fractures of varying ages evidenced by different stages of healing.

How would you treat this fracture?

I would treat this fracture in gallows traction with a radiograph at 2–3 weeks to show callus formation, and then gently mobilize as comfort allows. However, a hip spica could also be used as there is no significant shortening of the femur.

Viva 17

A 3-year-old child is referred from A&E with a 24-h history of fever, malaise, and reluctance to bear weight on his right leg.

What is your approach to this patient?

The A&E doctor has sent some routine bloods and organized an ultrasound scan of his right hip, which is shown above.

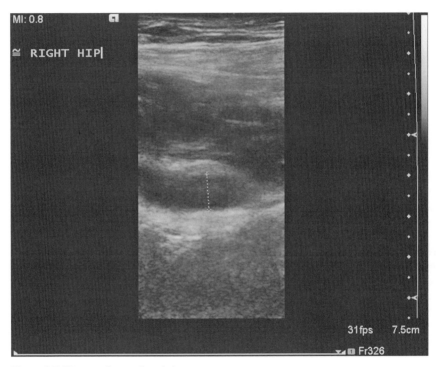

Figure 2.5 Ultrasound scan of a right hip.

How would you assess the child and what is your management now based on the hip scan?

What is your approach to this patient?

I would want to assess the child to exclude an infectious cause for his symptoms such as septic arthritis or osteomyelitis.

How would you assess the child and what is your management now based on the hip scan?

My clinical assessment would start with a detailed history from the parents.

On examination I would make an assessment of whether the child was well or unwell, and request basic observations including pulse, respiratory rate, and temperature. I would assess the resting posture and range of motion of the hips. I may find the hip to be in a position of most comfort (flexed, abducted, and externally rotated). I would also examine the whole lower limb, chest, abdomen, and spine.

The ultrasound shows an effusion around the right hip.

I would review the blood results and organize AP and lateral radiographs of clinically concerning areas to rule out any underlying structural abnormality or fracture.

The Kocher criteria can be used to help differentiate septic arthritis from transient synovitis:

1. Temperature > 38.5°C
2. White blood cells (WBC) > 12,000 cells/mm^3
3. ESR > 40 mm/h
4. Non-weight bearing on the affected side

The likelihood of septic arthritis increases with the number of positive factors present [1 = 3%, 2 = 40% (treat as septic arthritis), 3 = 93%, 4 = 99.6%]. A C-reactive protein (CRP) > 2.0 (mg/dl) is often also used as a positive predictor.

I would arrange an urgent aspiration of the hip joint and if this revealed pus, would proceed to an open washout of the hip as soon as possible (urgent case < 6 h).

I would approach the hip through an anterior approach and remove an ellipse of capsule to allow free drainage. I would take deep tissue samples for microbiology and perform copious washout with normal saline. I wouldn't routinely use a hip spica post-operatively but recognize there is a small risk of secondary subluxation and dysplasia. I would discuss appropriate antibiotic therapy with the microbiology team, usually starting with broad-spectrum intravenous antibiotics and then adjusting as guided by the culture results.

Daily orthopaedic review and serial inflammatory markers are necessary to ensure clinical improvement. The duration of antibiotic therapy is generally 3–6 weeks and can be administered orally once the clinical picture improves and sensitivities are known.

The child would also require longer-term follow-up to check the development and the growth of the hip joint.

Viva 18

You are asked to go and assess a newborn child on the maternity ward.

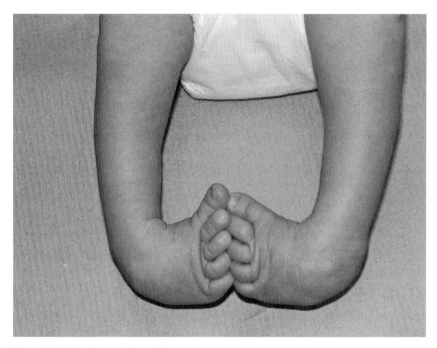

Figure 2.6 Clinical image of a newborn.

Describe the clinical photograph and the components of this deformity.

How do you classify the severity of this condition?

How would you take your management from here?

Describe the clinical photograph and the components of this deformity

This is a clinical photograph of a newborn child with a clubfoot deformity (congenital talipes equinovarus). This is a complex three-dimensional deformity seen at birth with midfoot cavus, fore-foot adductus, and hindfoot varus and equinus.

How do you classify the severity of this condition?

There are different scoring systems described to grade the severity of the deformity. In my institu-tion we use the Pirani scoring system. It comprises two parts, the midfoot contracture score (medial crease, curvature of lateral border, position of head of talus) and the hindfoot contracture score (posterior crease, empty heel, rigid equinus). Each individual component is graded 0, 0.5, or 1 to give a maximum total score of 6. A high score correlates to a more deformed foot.

How would you take your management from here?

I would manage this patient by taking a thorough history from the parents and examining the child to ensure they did not have any associated congenital anomalies or features to suggest that this might be a 'syndromic' clubfoot rather than an idiopathic clubfoot.

I would then explain and start the Ponseti serial casting method, which is now recognized world-wide as the gold-standard initial approach to clubfoot treatment.

The first key manoeuvre is to reduce the cavus deformity by dorsiflexing the first ray and unlocking the forefoot and midfoot. Elevation of the first ray produces supination, so I warn the parents the foot may look worse after the first cast. The second important manoeuvre is to abduct the forefoot at midfoot level using the uncovered head of the talus laterally as a fulcrum.

Above-knee casts (with the knee at 90°) are applied with moulding into the corrected position and then each week the old cast is removed, the foot is scored, and the next cast applied. The midfoot usually corrects well after four or five casts. If there is residual equinus (or < 20° of dorsiflexion) of the hindfoot, then an Achilles tenotomy can be performed under a local or GA. A final cast is applied in maximal dorsiflexion for a further 3 weeks while the tenotomy heals.

Infants then go into Denis Browne boots and bar (23 h/day for 3 months, then just at night and naptime until the age of 5 years). This holds the affected foot externally rotated at 70° and the normal foot at 40°. The vast majority of patients do very well, although compliance with the boots and bars can be an issue. Approximately 10–20% will require a tibialis anterior tendon transfer around the age of 4 for residual deformity or a dynamic in-toeing gait (supination of the foot during dorsiflexion).

Viva 19

Here is a child with cerebral palsy.

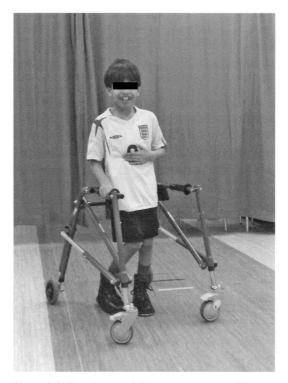

Figure 2.7 Clinical image of child with cerebral palsy/AP radiograph pelvis of child with cerebral palsy.

What is cerebral palsy and what different types do you know?

What is spasticity?

In what different ways do we manage spasticity?

Often ambulant children with cerebral palsy are assessed by gait analysis. What does that involve?

What is cerebral palsy and what different types do you know?

Cerebral palsy is a neuromuscular disorder caused by a non-progressive lesion to the immature developing brain (before the age of 2 years). Although the neurological injury is non-progressive, the musculoskeletal features evolve as the child grows.

Types of cerebral palsy are:

Anatomical—hemiplegia (40%)/diplegia (30%)/quadriplegic (30%)
Physiological—spastic (60%)/dystonic (20%)/ataxic (10%)/hypotonic (10%)
Functional—classified by the Gross Motor Function Classification System (GMFCS) I–V

What is spasticity?

Spasticity is a velocity-dependent increase in muscle tone causing resistance to movement.

In what different ways do we manage spasticity?

Principles include: a multidisciplinary approach involving family and patient in goal planning, decisions about treatments, and exploring expectations.

Non-operative treatment is based around a physiotherapist, who often acts as the main link between specialists. Adjuncts can be used to control spasticity including botulinum toxin injections and baclofen (tablets or intrathecal pump).

- Botulinum toxin A (derived from *Clostridium botulinum*) is injected locally (dose is weight dependent) into spastic muscles. It works by preventing release of acetylcholine at the neuromuscular junction of those tight muscles and is effective for 3–6 months. It is often used in combination with plasters/orthotics and targeted physiotherapy to maintain an improved stretch
- Baclofen is a gamma-aminobutyric acid (GABA) agonist (an inhibitory neurotransmitter), which acts both centrally and peripherally to decrease spasticity. If administered intrathecally, via an infusion pump, it allows an increased local dose with decreased systemic side-effects

Surgery is often needed, and appropriate planning and timing is crucial when performing multilevel surgery to avoid 'birthday syndrome'. Options can include bony surgery as well as soft-tissue procedures such as tenotomies, tendon lengthening, and tendon transfers.

Often ambulant children with cerebral palsy are assessed by gait analysis. What does that involve?

Gait analysis is the systematic description, assessment, and measurement of the components that characterize human locomotion. It involves the study of kinematics (the movements of individual body parts) and kinetics (the interaction of forces to produce those movements) as well as electromyography and energy consumption.

There is no defined standard; however, most gait laboratories will have two-dimensional video analysis and three-dimensional computer analysis, using specialized markers stuck onto specific bony landmarks. The computer program then breaks down the individual movements of anatomical parts into graphic form. Further detailed analysis involves the use of force plates, measuring ground reaction force, and electromyography, looking at muscle firing patterns.

It is important that the results of gait analysis are looked at in conjunction with a static detailed physical examination.

Viva 20

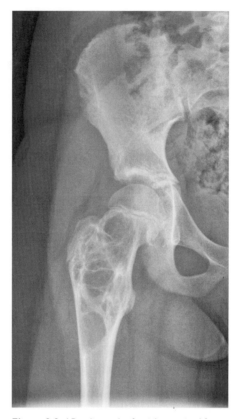

Figure 2.8 AP radiograph of a right proximal femur.

Can you describe the radiograph? What do you think the diagnosis is?

This patient presents with new-onset pain in the upper thigh. What do you think has happened?

How would you manage this patient now?

You treat expectantly, but unfortunately the lesion remains. How would you proceed now?

Can you describe the radiograph? What do you think the diagnosis is?

This is an AP radiograph showing a multiloculated lytic lesion in the left proximal femoral metaphysis of a skeletally immature individual. The zone of transition is sharp indicating this is likely to be a benign lesion, with no associated periosteal reaction or soft-tissue involvement. Top of my diagnosis would be a loculated simple bone cyst; however, an aneurysmal bone cyst is also a possibility.

This patient presents with new-onset pain in the upper thigh. What do you think has happened?

A lot of these lesions are found incidentally on radiographs taken for another reason, but new-onset pain in that area would suggest a pathological fracture through the weakened bone. A 'fallen leaf' sign (cortex that has fallen into the cystic cavity) is pathognomonic of this.

How would you manage this patient now?

Having taken a thorough history and examined the patient, I would probably manage this expectantly as in most cases the fracture stimulates new bone formation and over time the cyst fills in.

You treat expectantly, but unfortunately the lesion remains. How would you proceed now?

If an expectant, non-operative approach failed I would aspirate the cyst under image guidance and inject steroid and/or bone graft to try and stimulate new bone formation. If this failed, a repeated attempt is worthwhile; however, the definitive surgical treatment would involve curettage of the cyst through a small cortical window followed by stabilization of the bone to prevent fracture. If the cavity is close to the growth plate it is important not to damage it and risk growth arrest.

Viva 21

This 6-year-old child fell out of a tree onto their left arm.

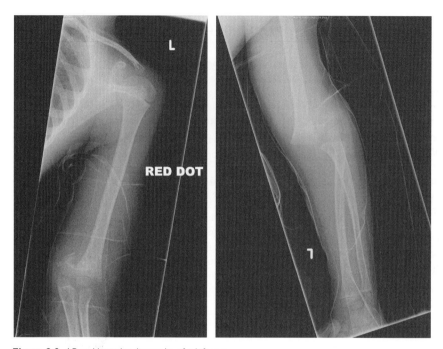

Figure 2.9 AP and lateral radiographs of a left arm.

Can you describe the radiograph?

How would you manage this child?

You reduce and pin the fracture under anaesthetic, but on post-operative review in recovery you are unable to feel a pulse. What would you do now?

Can you describe the radiograph?

There is an 'off-ended' Gartland 3 supracondylar fracture of the left distal humerus.

How would you manage this child?

Assuming this was an isolated injury I would assess the child for the presence of an open injury, and also assess the distal neurovascular status (colour of hand, capillary refill of the fingertips, radial pulse, sensation in the specific dermatomes, and motor function of ulnar, radial, median, and anterior interosseus nerves).

I would organize for the child to have analgesia and a temporary backslab splint to stop the arm from moving and then mobilize my theatre team, as this child needs to go to theatre as soon as possible for closed reduction and percutaneous pinning.

In theatre, the set-up of the image intensifier and the help of a good assistant is key. The technique for reduction is to apply good continuous traction (in 20° of flexion) for several minutes, then correct any valgus/varus and rotational deformity, before flexing up and hooking the distal fragment back on to the shaft. The forearm can be pronated to lock the fragments. I would insert a lateral wire first (2 mm), making sure I crossed the far cortex. With that wire offering some stability, it is possible to extend the arm slightly to perform a mini-open approach on the medial side, allowing protection of the ulna nerve while inserting the second wire. I would splint the arm in a backslab in near extension, reassess the perfusion of the hand, and monitor for compartment syndrome.

You reduce and pin the fracture under anaesthetic, but on post-operative review in recovery you are unable to feel a pulse. What would you do now?

If I could not feel a pulse, I would make an assessment of the general vascularity of the hand. If the hand was warm and pink, with adequate capillary refill, then I would monitor the situation with regular review. The artery is likely to be in spasm and the pulse can take a day or two to recover. If the hand was white and capillary refill reduced, I would release the backslab and allow the arm to extend to see if this improved the situation. If not, I would contact the vascular/plastic surgeons for an urgent review as the artery may have been caught up in the fracture and may now been occluded by the reduction. If so, this would require open exploration, usually via an anterior approach.

Viva 22

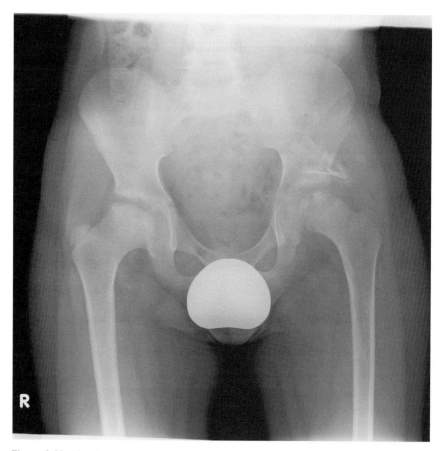

Figure 2.10 AP radiograph of a pelvis.

This radiograph shows a post-operative view of a boy's pelvis. What do you think the underlying diagnosis is and what procedure has he had?

What is the underlying disease and who gets it?

How do you classify this condition?

What are the principles of management?

This radiograph shows a post-operative view of a boy's pelvis. What do you think the underlying diagnosis is and what procedure has he had?

This is an AP pelvic radiograph of a skeletally immature patient showing flattening and deformity of both femoral heads in keeping with Perthes' disease (Legg–Calve–Perthes disease). On the left side this patient has had a shelf procedure, which is a salvage type of acetabular procedure. It is an operation that redistributes the weight-bearing load of the femoral head through a larger surface area of pelvic cover.

What is the underlying disease and who gets it?

Perthes' disease is idiopathic AVN of the proximal femoral epiphysis in childhood. It remains a controversial topic in orthopaedics because of its unknown aetiology and uncertain optimal treatment. It is more common in boys than girls by about 4:1 and it is bilateral in about 20% of cases.

How do you classify this condition?

There are many classifications used for Perthes' disease. Waldenström classified it into pathological stages:

1. Initial avascular event (crescent sign—representing a subchondral fracture)
2. Fragmentation (Herring's pillar classification)
3. Resolution—re-ossification
4. Remodelling—healed

The Herring classification of severity is based on the lateral pillar height on an AP radiograph during the fragmentation stage:

- B—more than 50% maintained
- C—less than 50% maintained

(A B/C border category was subsequently added.)
    Catterall's classification contains four groups depending on the amount of femoral head involved on the lateral radiograph.
    Catterall also added clinical and radiological 'head at risk signs', which he used to guide his management:

Clinical	Radiological
Obese	Horizontal physis
Progressive decreased ROM	Lateral subluxation of epiphysis
Abduction contracture	Lateral calcification
ER with flexion	Diffuse metaphyseal reaction
	Gage sign—inverted V-shaped lucency in lateral metaphysis

ROM, range of motion; ER, external rotation.

Stulberg's classification assessed the shape of femoral head at skeletal maturity and is used to predict who will do poorly in terms of early onset degenerative change:

I—normal
II—head spherical (magna/breva) and fits in socket, which is congruent
III—ovoid head (mushroom-shaped) congruent
IV—flat head and flat socket congruent
V—flat head incongruent

What are the principles of management?

Goals of treatment are:

1. Symptomatic relief
2. Containment of the head and hence correct development
3. Restoration of range of movement (ROM)

These goals can be achieved by various non-operative and operative treatments, which still are debated around the world.

Each patient should be managed on an individual basis taking into account their age, clinical signs, and radiological appearances on X-ray.

Viva 23

This 9 year old is undergoing treatment for genu valgum.

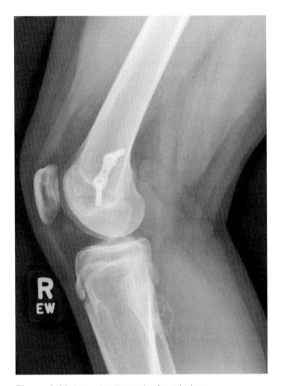

Figure 2.11 Lateral radiograph of a right knee.

Describe the radiograph.

What are the causes of genu valgum?

What factors are important to consider when planning such surgery?

Describe the radiograph

This is a lateral radiograph of a skeletally immature right knee with an eight plate *in situ* in the distal femur. The eight plate is a method of temporary hemiepiphysiodesis.

What are the causes of genu valgum?

Genu valgum is a normal physiological process and between the ages of 3 and 4 years, up to 20° of valgus deformity can be accepted. By the age of 7 years, more than 12° of valgus is considered pathological. Bilateral genu valgum can be caused by renal osteodystrophy or skeletal dysplasias, which include mucopolysaccharide storage diseases, such as Morquio syndrome. Unilateral genu valgum can occur secondary to physeal trauma, infection, infarction, or benign tumours such as osteochondromas.

What factors are important to consider when planning such surgery?

It is important to consider the age of the child and their potential for further growth. It is generally accepted that growth continues until 14 years in girls and 16 years in boys. Skeletal maturity can be estimated radiologically using bone age hand radiographs.

The distal femoral epiphysis is estimated to grow at 9 mm/year and the proximal tibia at 6 mm/year; however, regular follow-up is necessary to avoid overcorrection. Rebound deformity is not uncommon and this must also be taken into consideration.

Viva 24

This 10 year old presented with a shortened right limb and evidence of anteromedial bowing.

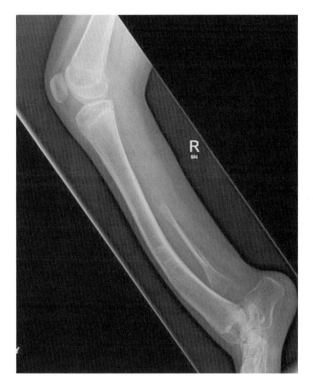

Figure 2.12 Lateral radiograph of a right lower leg.

Describe the radiograph.

What is the diagnosis and what other features might you look for?

What other types of tibial bowing are described in children?

Describe the radiograph

This is a lateral radiograph of the right lower limb in a skeletally immature child with anterior bowing of the tibia and absence of the proximal fibula.

What is the diagnosis and what other features might you look for?

The diagnosis is fibular hemimelia (otherwise known as fibular deficiency), which is the most common congenital long bone deficiency and can either present with shortening or entire absence of the fibula. Fibular hemimelia is a common cause of anteromedial bowing and often associated with cruciate ligament deficiencies. Tarsal coalitions occur in approximately 50% of patients, resulting in a ball and socket ankle joint that causes instability. Shortening of both the tibia and femur contribute to an overall leg length discrepancy and hypoplasia of the lateral femoral condyle can lead to genu valgum. Absent lateral rays are also a feature of the condition.

What other types of tibial bowing are described in children?

Posteromedial bowing is physiological and thought to be associated with intrauterine positioning. It can result in a leg length discrepancy of 3–4 cm, occasionally requiring epiphysiodesis.

Anterolateral bowing is pathological and associated with congenital pseudoarthrosis of the tibia and neurofibromatosis type I.

Part 2   **Basic Sciences**

Chapter 3 **Tissue Anatomy**

Viva 25

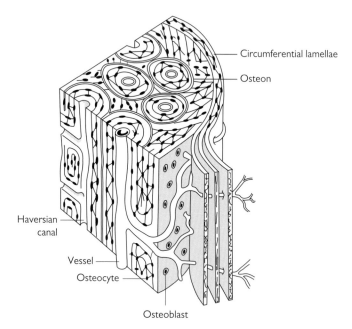

Circumferential lamellae

Osteon

Haversian canal

Vessel

Osteocyte

Osteoblast

Figure 3.1 A diagram of bone structure.

Reproduced from C. Bulstrode et al., *Oxford Textbook of Trauma and Orthopaedics* second edition, 2011, figure 1.3.10, p. 25, with permission from Oxford University Press.

What is bone?

How do osteoblasts and osteoclasts differ?

What is Wolff's law?

What is bone?

Bone is a composite dynamic form of specialized connective tissue.

It comprises cells (10%) and extracellular matrix (90%).

The cells include: osteoblasts, osteocytes, and osteoclasts.

The matrix has organic (collagens, mainly type 1) and inorganic (calcium phosphate, osteocalcium phosphate) constituents.

Bone functions to move, support, and protect the internal organs, it produces red and white blood cells, and contains the majority of calcium and phosphate in the body.

How do osteoblasts and osteoclasts differ?

Osteoblasts are derived from undifferentiated mesenchymal cells; they are bone forming and lay down osteoid (type 1 collagen) as well as activating osteoclasts to resorb bone via the receptor activator of nuclear factor kappa-B (RANK) ligand (RANKL) system. These processes are controlled by cytokines, growth factors, and bone morphogenic protein (BMP).

Osteoclasts are from a haemopoietic monocyte cell lineage. They are multinucleated giant cells that resorb bone. They can sit in small pits called Howship's lacunae, on the bone surface, or lead cutting cones that tunnel through the bone. Under their ruffled brush border, with an increased surface area, they create a low-pH microenvironment that dissolves the inorganic apatite crystals. Enzymes are released (tartrate-resistant acid phosphatase, TRAP) and proteases then break down the organic matrix components. This process is controlled via the RANKL system (inhibited by osteoprotegrin) of activated osteoblasts.

Osteocytes are osteoblasts that have become trapped in bone matrix (making up to 90% of the cells in bone). They have an important role in homeostasis of calcium and phosphate metabolism.

What is Wolff's law?

Wolff's law is a theory developed by the German anatomist/surgeon Julius Wolff in the 19th century. It states that bone will adapt to the loads placed through or across it. It is the result of the close coupling within bone remodelling units consisting of osteoblast, osteoclast, and supporting stromal tissues. If loading on a particular bone increases, the bone will remodel itself over time to become stronger to resist that sort of loading.

In relation to soft tissue, Davis's law explains how soft tissue remoulds itself according to imposed demands.

Viva 26

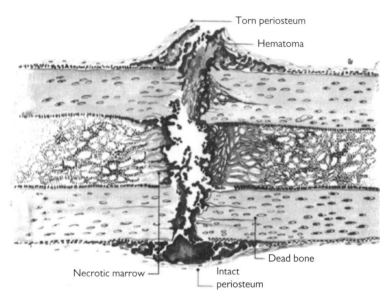

Torn periosteum

Hematoma

Dead bone

Necrotic marrow

Intact periosteum

Figure 3.2 A diagram of a fracture healing.

Reproduced from Cruess, R., and Dumont, J., Fracture healing, *Canadian Journal of Surgery*, 18, pp. 403–413, 1975, © Canadian Medical Association. This work is protected by copyright and the making of this copy was with the permission of Access Copyright. Any alteration of its content or further copying in any form whatsoever is strictly prohibited unless otherwise permitted by law.

Tell me how bones unite after a fracture.

What is the difference between intramembranous and endochondral ossification?

How do bones get wider?

Tell me how bones unite after a fracture

Secondary fracture healing can be divided into five stages: haematoma, inflammatory reaction, soft callus formation, hard callus formation, and remodelling; however, in reality these stages merge into a continuum.

Haematoma (hours)

The damage to tissue surfaces and blood vessels results in vasoconstriction and haematoma formation—platelet plugs form and the activated platelets degranulate releasing platelet-derived growth factor (PDGF). The clotting cascade and the complement system are both activated—these are stepwise amplification cascades that result in the activation of cytokines and signalling molecules which are chemotactic to the inflammatory cells and angiogenic to blood vessels. Released opsonins attach to bacteria and dead necrotic cells to expedite their phagocytosis. BMPs (BMP 7 is important) are also released from damaged bone straight away; they are osteoinductive, mitogenic, and angiogenic.

Inflammatory phase (days)

The arrival and activation of polymorph neutrophils (which also release activated cytokines and leukotrienes) is the start of the inflammatory phase. A bit later the next cells to arrive are the macrophages, which start to phagocytose dead cells and tissue.

Angiogenesis has started and helps to bring in new undifferentiated mesenchymal cells.

Repair phase—soft to hard callus (weeks)

The end of the inflammatory phase occurs with the arrival of fibroblasts and the beginning of the repair phase.

This phase can be thought of with regard to:

1. The mechanical environment, which delineates which cells form from the undifferentiated mesenchymal cells
2. The biochemical environment (oxygen tension and pH). Haematoma is acidic—osteoblasts need an alkaline environment to lay down bone

A fracture gap strain of 10–100% promotes fibroblast proliferation—fibrous tissue forms in the fracture gap and it becomes less mobile (angiogenesis continues). With a strain of < 10% chondrocytes proliferate, laying down collagen matrix and soft callus in the fracture gap. With < 2% strain the osteoblasts start to lay down osteoid, which is then mineralized to form hard callus (woven bone).

Remodelling phase (months to years)

The last phase, which lasts many months, is remodelling, where disorganized woven bone is stress orientated into hard dense lamellar bone (obeying the mechanical principles of Wolff's law).

What is the difference between intramembranous and endochondral ossification?

Endochondral ossification is the process associated with foetal bone development, day-to-day bone growth, and to a certain extent fracture repair. The replacement of cartilage by bone is called endochondral ossification. This is the type of bone formation found in the development of long bones such as the femur and humerus.

Intramembranous ossification is the formation of bone on, or in, fibrous connective tissue (which is formed from condensed mesenchyme cells). Intramembraneous ossification is the process used to make flat bones such as the mandible and flat bones of the skull.

How do bones get wider?

The increase in diameter is called appositional growth. Osteoblasts in the periosteum form compact bone around the external bone surface. At the same time, osteoclasts in the endosteum break down bone on the internal bone surface, around the medullary cavity. These two processes together increase the diameter of the bone.

Viva 27

A   B   C

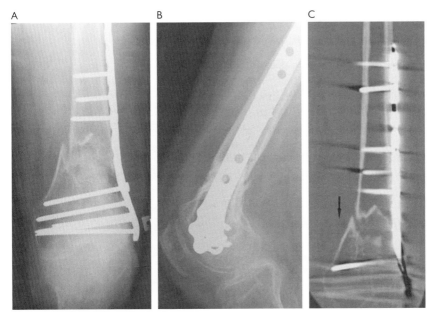

Figure 3.3 Radiographs of distal femoral fracture fixation.

This patient fractured a femur 4 months ago, but is still getting significant pain. What do you see and how would you manage it?

What factors influence fracture healing?

This patient fractured a femur 4 months ago, but is still getting significant pain. What do you see and how would you manage it?

This is an antero-posterior (AP) radiograph showing a supracondylar fracture of the femur treated with a locking plate device. The fracture doesn't show any signs of healing and at 4 months post-fixation this would be an established non-union.

I would approach this fracture using the following principles (5 S's):

Sepsis—first infection must be excluded as this can also cause non-union

Straighten—restore alignment

Stabilize—absolute versus relative stability construct

Stimulate—consider bone graft (autologous vs allograft vs BMP)

Soft tissue—ensure adequate soft-tissue cover

What factors influence fracture healing?

1. Fracture mechanical environment
2. Local biology
   Blood supply
   Degree of soft-tissue injury
   Open or closed injury
   Degree of fragmentation/bone loss
   Site of fracture (metaphyseal versus diaphyseal)
   Soft-tissue interposition
   Stability (cf. absolute/relative/dynamization)
   Presence of infection
   Presence of pathological lesion
   Previous irradiation to that area
3. Systemic biology
   Age
   Smoking
   Drugs—non-steroidal anti-inflammatory drugs (NSAIDs), steroids, bisphosphonates
   Medical co-morbidities—diabetes mellitus (DM)
   Nutrition
   Associated head injury

Viva 28

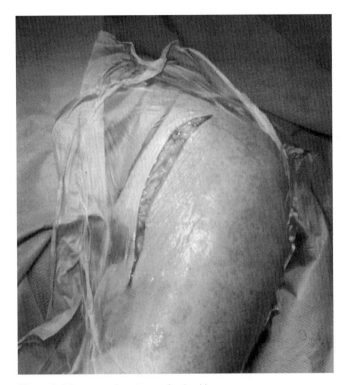

Figure 3.4 Intraoperative picture of a shoulder.
Reproduced from C. Bulstrode et al., *Oxford Textbook of Trauma and Orthopaedics* second edition, 2011, figure 4.9.4, p. 340, with permission from Oxford University Press.

Can you describe the deltopectoral approach to the glenohumeral joint?

Can you describe the patient set-up, primary, and secondary portals for ankle arthroscopy?

Can you describe the deltopectoral approach to the glenohumeral joint?

NB: You should be able do the same thing for all common approaches.

In an appropriately consented and marked patient, under general anaesthetic (GA) ± interscalene block, I would prepare them in a beach chair position.

Incision is from 1–2 cm inferior to the tip of the coracoid process extending towards the anterior axillary fold. The deltopectoral groove is identified by a 'yellow stripe' of fat and the cephalic vein is sought lying in the groove. The vein is usually reflected laterally.

The interval between the deltoid and the pectoralis major is developed and the conjoined tendon arising from the coracoid process is identified. The conjoined tendon is now dissected free from the underlying subscapularis. The conjoined tendon is retracted medially with the help of the self-retaining retractors (± partial division 1 cm distal to the coracoid). The subscapularis muscle and its tendon are identified by externally rotating the arm. Stay sutures are used to control the medial musculotendinous tissues of the subscapularis. With the arm in external rotation (ER), division of the subscapularis tendon is carried out about 1–2 cm from its insertion just lateral to the musculotendinous junction. Depending on indication, the subscapularis muscle is then either stripped off the anterior capsule or the capsule is divided with the tendon.

Nerves at risk

- The axillary nerve lies just inferior to the shoulder joint capsule. A blunt ring-handled retractor is slipped down on the anterior capsule and passed inferior to the shoulder, retracting the inferior structures including the axillary nerve away from the capsule, thereby protecting this important nerve, which lies only 5–10 mm below the inferior capsular fold
- The musculocutaneous nerve

Can you describe the patient set-up, primary, and secondary portals for ankle arthroscopy?

Pre-operatively I would mark the course of the superficial perineal nerve.

In an appropriately consented and marked patient, supine on the operating table under GA and a thigh tourniquet set to 300mmHg, I would set up using a bolster behind the thigh followed by longitudinal traction using a well-padded ankle distractor.

Ankle portals

1. Anteromedial: initial arthroscopy is performed with the scope in the anteromedial portal, but for the majority of cases this portal will be used for instrumentation, located at the level of the ankle joint, just medial to the tibialis anterior tendon, and located about 5 mm lateral to the medial malleolus. An 18-gauge syringe is used to infuse saline into the joint; the greater saphenous nerve and vein are at risk with this portal, lying 7–9 mm medial to the portal
2. Anterolateral: once the joint is distended with saline, use an 18-gauge needle to mark the location of the anterolateral portal, which should lie just lateral to the peroneus tertius tendon; staying lateral to the peroneus tertius helps avoid injury to the dorsal lateral branch of the peroneal nerve. Use the scope to transilluminate the anterolateral skin, in order to look for underlying cutaneous nerves; the scope can then be driven forward (elevating the synovium and skin), which further assists with placement of this portal. Make a small incision and then spread with a haemostat; be aware that the intermediate branch of the superficial peroneal nerve is about 5–6 mm from this portal

NB: You should be able to do the same thing for the knee and the shoulder.

Viva 29

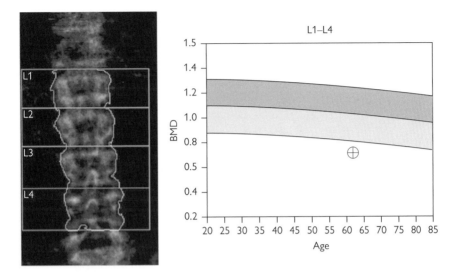

Results Summary:

Region	Area[cm²]	BMC[(g)]	BMD[(g/cm²)]	T-score	PR (Peak Reference)	Z-score	AM (Age Matched)
L1	17.25	13.34	0.773	−2.7	72	−2.1	77
L2	17.89	12.60	0.746	−3.2	68	−2.5	73
L3	17.72	12.64	0.713	−3.5	65	−2.9	69
L4	18.84	11.87	0.630	−4.2	58	−3.5	62
Total	70.70	50.45	0.714	−3.4	65	−2.8	70

Figure 3.5 A picture of an imaging modality.

Reproduced from Raashid Luqmani, Theodore Pincus, and Maarten Boers, *Rheumatoid Arthritis* (Oxford Rheumatology Library), 2010, Figure 8.2, p. 84, with permission from Oxford University Press.

What investigation is illustrated above?

Define osteoporosis and list its risk factors.

What numerical results are given by this test and how do you interpret them?

Can you describe the treatment of osteoporosis, the drugs, and how they act?

What investigation is illustrated above?

A bone-density scan.

Define osteoporosis and list its risk factors

Osteoporosis is a condition in which decreased bone mineral density results in increased susceptibility to low-trauma fragility fractures.

Osteoporosis (in women) is defined by the World Health Organization as a bone mineral density 2.5 standard deviations (SD) below peak bone mass (20-year-old healthy female average) as measured on a dual-energy X-ray absorptiometry (DEXA) scan.

Risk factors for osteoporosis include:

- Low-impact fracture
- New thoracic kyphosis
- Early menopause < 48 years [oestrogen blocks the effect of parathyroid hormone (PTH) on osteoclasts]
- Family history of hip or vertebral fracture in first-degree relative < 65 years old
- Predisposing pathology: hypothyroid, rheumatoid arthritis, alcohol, Cushing's, malignancy
- Prolonged amenorrhoea in the absence of pregnancy
- Drugs: steroids, thyroxine, heparin, phenytoin, chemotherapy

What numerical results are given by this test and how do you interpret them?

Really, there are only four important numbers, and two of these are of lesser importance:

1. First, identify the percentage of normal bone density for the patient's age. This is helpful in your explanation to patients, but doesn't really affect diagnosis or treatment (this is one of the numbers you can ignore if you wish)
2. Second, find the Z-score, which is the SD from normal for that patient's age group (this is the other number you can ignore)
3. Third, find the percentage of bone density compared with normal young adults. This number has a powerful impact on patients. Ninety per cent and above is considered normal. It is important to tell patients that this is the amount of bone that they *have* compared to what they *had* or *should have had* at the age of 40
4. Fourth, find the T-score, which is the number of SD from normal young adults. *This is the key number* as it is from this that the World Health Organization takes its *definition of osteoporosis.* The T-score shows where your patient is compared with the population. In other words, an Irish woman with a small frame stacks up differently from an African American woman with a larger frame, and you want to know how they compare with people of their own sex, race, age, height, and weight. The T-score predicts fracture risk: for every −1 SD the fracture risk doubles. Osteoporosis is defined as a T-score > 2.5 SD below mean (lumbar spine) [the bone mineral density (BMD) of a fit and healthy 25 year old]

Can you describe the treatment of osteoporosis, the drugs, and how they act?

Treatment guidelines from the National Institute of Health and Clinical Excellence (NICE) are divided into lifestyle changes and pharmacological treatment.

All at-risk patients and those with confirmed osteoporosis (either by fracture or DEXA scan) should have information regarding lifestyle changes, which include: taking weight-bearing exercise, reducing alcohol consumption, stopping smoking, and reducing falls risk.

All patients should have calcium (1500 mg) and vitamin D (800 IU) supplements.

Female patients who are post-menopausal < 65 years old with T-score > 3 or > 75 years old with osteoporotic fracture should have:

- First-line treatment—bisphosphonates. Alendronate 70 mg once a week
- Second-line treatment—strontium ranelate 2 mg once daily (may affect future DEXA scans)
- Third-line treatment—raloxifene 60 mg once daily

Bisphosphonates are the main pharmacological measures for treatment. They work by inhibiting osteoclast function and hence resorption of bone. They attach to the osteoclast and prevent the attachment of its ruffled brush border to the bone.

Strontium ranelate stimulates proliferation of the osteoblasts, as well as inhibiting the proliferation of osteoclasts.

Raloxifene is a selective oestrogen receptor modulator. It works by attaching itself to oestrogen receptors in the bone, stimulating the production of new bone.

Three key elements of a strategy for osteoporotic fractures are:

1. High-quality fracture care—delivered through coordinated multidisciplinary teamwork
2. High-quality secondary prevention of fragility fracture—ensured by providing bone protection and falls assessment
3. High-quality information—using standards, audit, and feedback to improve hip fracture care and secondary prevention

NB: osteopenia = T-score –2.5 to –1.0. Treat with lifestyle changes only.

Viva 30

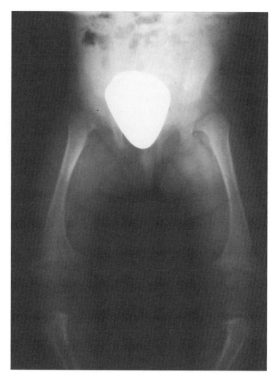

Figure 3.6 A radiograph of a skeletally immature patient.

Reproduced from David A. Warrell, Timothy M. Cox, and John D. Firth, *Oxford Textbook of Medicine* fifth edition, 2010, figure 20.1.9, p. 3737, with permission from Oxford University Press.

The radiograph above was performed on a child who presented with bowed legs.

What do you think the diagnosis is?

What is rickets?

What are the causes of rickets?

How else might a child with rickets present, and how would you investigate them?

What do you think the diagnosis is?

This plain radiograph of the pelvis and knees shows generalized widening of the metaphysis and cupping of the epiphysis in keeping with a metabolic condition such as rickets. Differential diagnosis would include a generalized skeletal dysplasia.

What is rickets?

Rickets is a disease of growing bone that is unique to children and adolescents. It is caused by a failure of osteoid to calcify in a growing person. Failure of osteoid to calcify in adults is called osteomalacia.

What are the causes of rickets?

Familial hypophosphataemic rickets (vitamin D resistant)
Vitamin D resistance (type I and type II)
Vitamin D deficient (nutritional rickets)
Renal osteodystrophy
Hypophosphatasia

How else might a child with rickets present, and how would you investigate them?

The child may present with generalized muscular hypotonia of an unknown mechanism. In the long bones, laying down of uncalcified osteoid at the metaphyses leads to spreading of those areas, producing knobby deformity that is visualized on radiography as cupping and flaring of the metaphyses. Weight bearing produces deformities such as bowlegs and knock-knees. In the chest, knobbly deformities result in the rachitic rosary along the costochondral junctions. The weakened ribs pulled by muscles also produce flaring over the diaphragm, which is known as the Harrison groove. The sternum may be pulled into a pigeon-breast deformity. At the ankle, palpation of the tibial malleolus gives the impression of a double epiphysis (Marfan's sign).

Blood tests

Early on in the disease course, the calcium (ionized fraction) is low; however, it is often within the reference range at the time of diagnosis as PTH levels increase. Calcidiol (25-hydroxy vitamin D) levels are low, and PTH levels are elevated; however, determining calcidiol and PTH levels is typically not necessary. Alkaline phosphatase levels are elevated.

Viva 31

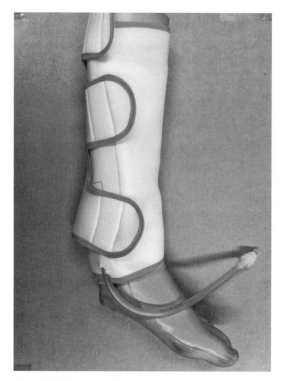

Figure 3.7 An image of a clinical device.

Do you use this device in your clinical practice?

Describe Virchow's triad and the risk factors for formation of a deep vein thrombosis (DVT).

What risk levels do you quote to patients undergoing total hip replacement (THR) and total knee replacement (TKR)?

What is your DVT prophylaxis policy for THR in a 70-year-old man with no significant additional risk factors?

Do you use this device in your clinical practice?

Yes, this is a mechanical calf pump that we use intra-operatively to prevent venous thrombosis.

Describe Virchow's triad and the risk factors for formation of a deep vein thrombosis (DVT)

Virchow's triad includes:

1. Hypercoagulable state
2. Stasis of vascular flow
3. Damage to the vascular endothelium

What risk levels do you quote to patients undergoing total hip replacement (THR) and total knee replacement (TKR)?

Forty to 60% of THR patients who do not receive prophylaxis will get a DVT (dependent on imaging method). With chemical and mechanical prophylaxis asymptomatic DVT occurs in 10% of THR and 20% of TKR patients. Symptomatic DVT occurs in 1.3% of TKR patients and 2.81% of THR patients.

What is your DVT prophylaxis policy for THR in a 70-year-old man with no significant additional risk factors?

The two main strategies for prevention are:

1. Non-pharmacological interventions. These include anti-DVT stockings and foot or calf pumps
2. Pharmacological interventions. These include one or more of the following:
   - Low-molecular-weight heparin (LMWH): heparin and LMWH are equivalent in preventing DVT, although LMWH has greater bioavailability, longer duration of anticoagulant effect in fixed doses, and little requirement for laboratory monitoring, and is thus more cost-effective
   - Fondaparinux sodium: a synthetic pentasaccharide. When used at 2.5 mg subcutaneously (SC) four times a day post-operatively, it significantly improves the risk-to-benefit ratio for the prevention of post-operative venous thromboembolism
   - Warfarin: an effective but cumbersome DVT prophylaxis regimen is achieved with either a fixed or an adjusted dose
   - Rivaroxaban: like Fondaparinux, this is a Factor Xa inhibitor, but is taken orally, in a once-a-day regime
   - Aspirin: however, there is not much evidence of its efficacy

You should be able to quote your local policy on what they use in this situation.

Viva 32

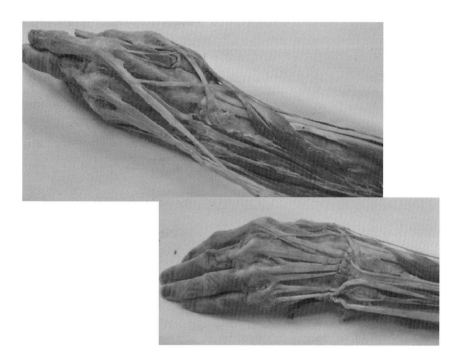

Figure 3.8 A diagram of the forearm.

Reproduced with permission from MacKinnon P, Morris J. (2005). *Oxford Textbook of Functional Anatomy*, Vol. 1. Oxford: Oxford University Press, © 2005.

Can you tell me about the organization of extensor tendons at the wrist?

Can you give me an example of pathology in any of the compartments?

What are the principles of tendon transfer?

Can you tell me about the organization of extensor tendons at the wrist?

There are six extensor compartments numbered from radial to ulnar on the dorsum of the wrist.

1 Extensor pollicis brevis, abductor pollicis longus
2 Extensor carpi radialis longus, extensor carpi radialis brevis
3 Extensor pollicis longus
4 Extensor indicis proprius, extensor digitorum communis, posterior interosseus nerve
5 Extensor digiti minimi
6 Extensor carpi ulnaris

Can you give me an example of pathology in any of the compartments?

1 de Quervain's synovitis
2 Intersection syndrome
3 Drummer's wrist
4 Extensor tenosynovitis
5 Vaughan Jackson syndrome
6 Extensor carpi ulnaris (ECU) snapping

What are the principles of tendon transfer?

- Power—should ideally 5/5 prior to transfer—as a general rule each transferred tendon will lose one unit of power
- Range—of movement
- Out—an expendable tendon
- Function—one tendon = one movement
- Excursion—adequate displacement of tendon is possible in the transferred position
- Synergistic
- Straight line of pull

Mnemonic PROFESS

I would only perform tendon transfers in a motivated patient with the capacity for rehabilitation and where the surgeon is part of multidisciplinary team including hand therapists and occupational therapists.

Viva 33

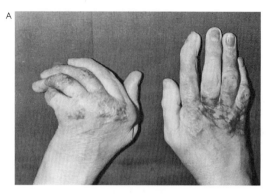

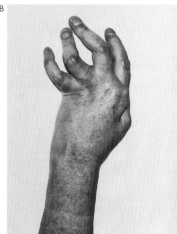

Figure 3.9 A picture of a patient's hands.

Reproduced from C. Bulstrode et al., *Oxford Textbook of Trauma and Orthopaedics* second edition, 2011, figure 6.5.1, p. 447, with permission from Oxford University Press.

What do you understand by the term rheumatoid arthritis?

How does one diagnose rheumatoid arthritis?

Can you tell me anything about the aetiology of rheumatoid arthritis?

Clinically, how does it manifest itself?

What are the X-ray features that distinguish rheumatoid from osteoarthritis?

What are your principles for managing a patient with rheumatoid arthritis?

What do you understand by the term rheumatoid arthritis?

Rheumatoid arthritis is a T-cell mediated inflammatory disease that has both systemic and joint manifestations. Classically there is an erosive deforming symmetrical arthritis affecting large and small joints.

How does one diagnose rheumatoid arthritis?

This is performed using a scoring system outlined by the American College of Rheumatologists. Key features in the diagnosis are in four domains:

1. Joint involvement (large and small)
2. Serology [rheumatoid factor and anti-cyclic citrullinated peptides (CCP)]
3. Acute phase reactants [C-reactive protein (CRP) and erythrocyte sedimentation rate (ESR)]
4. Duration of symptoms (> 6 weeks)

Can you tell me anything about the aetiology of rheumatoid rrthritis?

There is a progressive inflammatory response seen against cartilage, bone, and soft tissues. Commonly antigen-presenting cells, T helper, NK, plasma. HLA DR4 and HLA DW4 cofactors are seen that activate collagenases and proteases. These in turn cause cartilage and peri-articular capsulo-ligamentous attenuation.

Clinically, how does it manifest itself?

This can be described as occurring within joints and systemically. Joint problems are typically morning stiffness, pain, and symmetrical swelling. It is associated with carpal tunnel syndrome and Vaughan Jackson syndrome. Extra-articular involvement includes: ocular inflammation, amyloidosis, nephropathy, cardiac, pleurisy, neuropathy, nodules, Flety's syndrome, Sjogren's syndrome, and the anaemia of chronic disease.

What are the X-ray features that distinguish rheumatoid from osteoarthritis?

Osteoarthritis	rheumatoid arthritis
Joint space narrowing	Joint space narrowing
Deformity and malalignment	N/A
Cysts	Erosions
Sclerosis	Osteoporosis
Osteophytes	N/A
Loose bodies	N/A
Asymmetrical	Symmetrical
Normal soft tissue	Soft-tissue contractures

What are your principles for managing a patient with rheumatoid arthritis?

Control synovitis and inflammation—rest/splint/anti-inflammatories/disease-modifying anti-rheumatic drugs (DMARDS) (biological and non-biological)

Maintain joint function—DMARDS, physiotherapy, surgery

Prevent deformity—physiotherapy +/− tendon reconstruction or transfer

Reconstruction—excision arthroplasty/arthroplasty

Viva 34

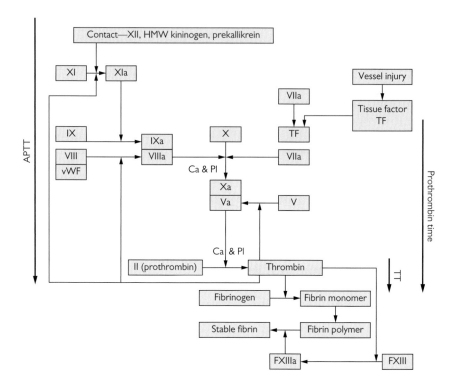

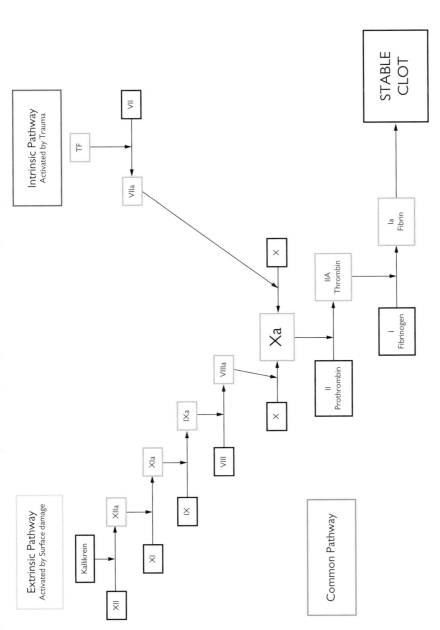

Figure 3.10 A schematic of the clotting cascade.

Reproduced from R. Leach et al., *Oxford Desk Reference Acute Medicine*, 2016, figure 12.2, p. 534, with permission from Oxford University Press.

What do you understand about the process of haemostasis in the normal patient?

Do you know of any hypercoagulable states?

Do you know of any haematological diseases that predispose to bleeding?

Do you know of any medications that are used to alter the clotting potential of blood in the medical setting?

What do you understand about the process of haemostasis in the normal patient?

Haemostasis is the normal physiological process by which the body responds to blood vessel injury and bleeding. Its purpose is to minimize blood loss, temporarily repair a blood vessel, and provide a framework for tissue repair.

It can be divided into primary and secondary haemostasis.

In primary haemostasis a platelet plug is formed. Damage to the endothelial cell leads to the exposure of collagen. von Willebrands factor (vWF) attaches to the exposed collagen. Platelets have receptors for vWF called GP1b and these lead to the indirect adhesion of the platelet to the vessel wall. Adhesion of the platelet leads to its activation and the release of granule contents such as ADP, calcium, serotonin, and thromboxane A2 (TXA2). The platelet also upregulates its expression of Gp2b and Gp3a receptors. This initiates further platelets to adhere and a feedback loop establishes, promoting the production of a primary platelet plug.

In secondary haemostasis, there is the formation of an insoluble cross-linked fibrin plug by activated coagulation factors, the most important of which is thrombin. The fibrin stabilizes the primary platelet plug particularly in larger blood vessels where the platelet plug alone is insufficient to stop haemorrhage.

Secondary haemostasis was originally explained via the cascade system, which was proposed in 1964. More recently, it has become accepted that the cell-based model, which focuses on the interaction between tissue factor-bearing cells and platelets, more accurately represents the process that occurs *in vivo*. The cell-based model describes three independent but overlapping steps: initiation, amplification, and propagation.

The cascade system however remains useful as it is important for the interpretation of laboratory results and demonstrates how coagulation works in the *in vitro* setting.

The cascade system is divided into the intrinsic (contact activation) and the extrinsic (tissue factor) pathway. The extrinsic pathway is shorter and more clinically significant; however, it is important to recognize that if a defect is present in one pathway the other cannot compensate. Both pathways must be functioning for normal haemostasis to occur.

Both the intrinsic and extrinsic pathways lead to the activation of factor X. The common pathway leads to the production of fibrin and a stable clot. The intrinsic pathway activity is measured by activated partial thromboplastin time (APTT) and the extrinsic pathway by international normalized ratio (INR).

A summary of this process is shown in Figure 3.10.

Do you know of any hypercoagulable states?

Yes. These include: factor V Leiden thrombophilia, antithrombin III deficiency, protein S and protein C deficiency.

Do you know of any haematological diseases that predispose to bleeding?

Yes. These include: von Willebrand disease, haemophilia A (an X-linked recessive condition caused by factor VIII deficiency), and haemophilia B (an X-linked recessive condition caused by factor IX deficiency. Haemophilia B is also known as Christmas disease, named for Stephen Christmas, the first patient in whom this condition was identified. He worked as a hospital photographer and campaigner for transfusion safety. He died of the complications of AIDS in 1993 as a result of the multiple blood transfusions he received over his lifetime).

Do you know of any medications that are used to alter the clotting potential of blood in the medical setting?

Yes. These include:

Warfarin. A coumarin that acts to inhibit the vitamin K-dependent synthesis of factors II, VII, XI, and X. It has a half-life of 40 h and is monitored by the INR. It should be stopped 5 days before surgery. It is reversed by the use of vitamin K or fresh frozen plasma (FFP) and is not safe for use in pregnancy

Heparin. This is a cofactor for the activation of antithrombin. Antithrombin acts to inhibit factors IIa, VII, IX, XI, and XII. It has a quick onset and a half-life of only 1 h. It needs to be stopped a minimum of 3 h before surgery. It can be reversed with protamine

LMWH. This acts primarily to inhibit the activation of factor Xa. It has a longer half-life than heparin (4 h) and a greater bioavailability. It needs to be stopped at least 24 h prior to surgery and cannot be reversed with protamine. It is administered subcutaneously

Fondaparinux (rivoroxaban). This is a synthetic factor Xa inhibitor. It has a half-life of 8–12 h and can be taken orally

Aspirin. Acts to inhibit TXA2 production in platelets, a proaggregation factor. Although its half-life is only 20 min, its effect on platelets is irreversible

Clopidogrel. Binds irreversibly to ADP receptors on platelets to prevent platelet aggregation. It has a half-life of 8 h but owing to its irreversible nature must be stopped 7 days prior to surgery

Chapter 4   **Mechanics and Tribology**

Viva 35

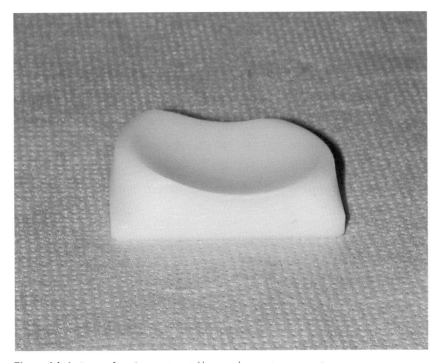

Figure 4.1 An image of a unicompartmental knee replacement component.

What is this material?

How is it manufactured?

How can its material properties be manipulated?

What is this material?

This is an ultra-high-molecular-weight polyethylene (UHMWPE) component from a unicompartmental knee replacement. UHMWPE is a long hydrocarbon chain held together by covalent bonds. The chain exists in two phases: a disorganized amorphous phase and a more organized crystalline phase. Three types are available (GUR 1020, 1050, 1090), which have increasing molecular weight.

How is it manufactured?

It is manufactured using the Zeigler process as follows:

1. Ethylene gas is polymerized in a low-temperature, low-pressure environment. The catalyst used is titanium chloride. This produces a fine UHMWPE powder
2. The UHMWPE powder is then processed by one of the following methods:
   Ram extrusion: produces bar stock, lowest quality
   Sheet compression moulding: higher quality
   Direct compression moulding (e.g. Arcom by Biomet): the UHMWPE powder is moulded into the shape of the final component. Better quality control, but expensive
3. Machining: UHMWPE bar, sheets, or moulded components are shaped into their final form
4. Sterilization and packaging: by gamma irradiation, gas plasma, or ethylene oxide

How can its material properties be manipulated?

By making cross-linked polyethylene (XLPE).

The manufacture of XLPE involves bombarding the material with an electron beam or gamma irradiation, which causes chain scission of double covalent bonds, followed by rebonding, either by oxidation or cross-linking between adjacent polymer chains. To prevent oxidation owing to the formation of free radicals, the process is performed in an inert environment (a vacuum or noble gas). XLPE must be annealed, to release oxygen free radicals from the material, as they will cause slow oxidation and therefore reduce shelf life. Some manufacturers add antioxidants (e.g. vitamin E).

- Advantages of XLPE are: 80–100% reduction of *in vivo* wear
- Disadvantages of XLPE are: it is more brittle and therefore at increased risk of fracture (there is debate as to whether it is suitable for use in the knee)

Viva 36

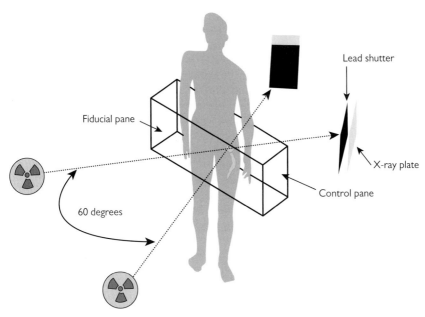

Figure 4.2 An imaging schematic.

What is shown in this picture?

How does it work?

What is it used for?

What is shown in this picture?

A Roentgen stereophotogrammetric analysis (RSA).

How does it work?

RSA is a method for determining the three-dimensional coordinates of an object within the calibration cage, from two two-dimensional X-ray images. Tantalum marker beads are inserted into bone at the time of surgery. Post-operatively, the subject is placed within the calibration cage, which contains tantalum marker beads placed at accurately measured points. Two X-ray sources are placed at a known angle to each other. Stereo X-ray images are then taken simultaneously. The distance between the X-ray sources and the calibration cage is known; therefore, the three-dimensional coordinates of any point on the two-dimensional stereo X-ray images can be determined.

What is it used for?

RSA is predominantly used to measure the 'migration', over time, of joint replacements. It is used as a surrogate measure of outcome and has been shown to be an accurate predictor of failure in total hip arthroplasty. Most joint replacements migrate during the first 2 years of implantation. If there is rapid, sustained migration during this period, then there is an increased risk of failure. RSA is therefore a useful tool for evaluating new designs of joint replacement. The technique has a high statistical power implying that only about 20 patients are required per study, which typically takes 2 years to complete. The direction of migration of stems is clinically relevant and is design-dependent. For example, when an Exeter stem has 1.5 mm of distal migration, this is not associated with an increased risk of failure. Conversely, a distal migration of 1.5 mm in the Charnley Elite stem is associated with a 30% failure rate at 8 years.

Viva 37

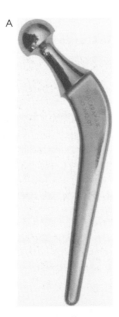

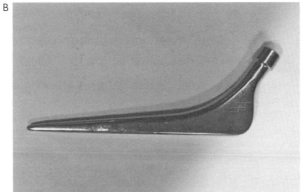

Figure 4.3 Two cemented hip stems.
Photograph courtesy of Paul Cooper

What are these devices?

What are the characteristic features of these designs?

Tell me about their design philosophy? How do they work?

How do they fail?

What are these devices?

These are two cemented stems. The first is an evolution of the Charnley stem; the second is the Exeter stem.

What are the characteristic features of these designs?

The Charnley-type stem is an example of a composite beam design, which has a collar or flange and a non-polished surface finish.

The Exeter is an example of a polished, double-tapered stem.

Tell me about their design philosophy? How do they work?

The composite beam or 'shape-closed' design philosophy relies on friction to maintain the position of the stem within the cement mantle. A rough surface finish (typically greater than 2 Ra) and design features, such as a collar or flange, are intended to minimize micromotion at the prosthesis–cement interface. The Exeter stem works on the taper slip (or force-closed) principle, whereby stability is achieved by allowing micromovement at the prosthesis–cement interface. These devices have design features that promote migration; these include a collarless geometry and a highly polished surface finish (< 0.01 Ra). Polished, tapered stems subside within the cement mantle, and in so doing they generate radial stresses that increase compression at the bone–cement and prosthesis–cement interfaces. In turn, this stabilizes the bone–cement–prosthesis composite. The viscoelastic properties of cement (creep and stress relaxation) are a key factor in this process.

How do they fail?

Common causes of failure of hip implants are infection, trauma, and specific causes secondary to design features.

In terms of cement fixation failure, composite beam stems fail when movement occurs at the prosthesis–cement interface. A rough surface finish will abrade the cement mantle once micromovement is established. This probably leads to gap formation, which in turn further increases micromovement and also allows the circulation of wear debris. Polished, tapered stems are inherently stable devices and their mechanism of failure is not well understood. RSA and retrieval studies suggest that these devices fail when they rotate in the axial plane.

Viva 38

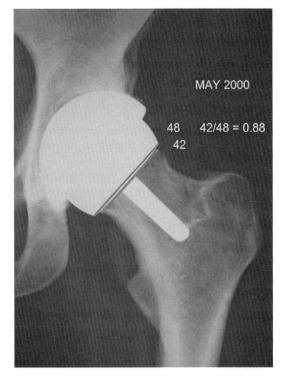

MAY 2000

48   42/48 = 0.88
42

Figure 4.4 A post-operative AP radiograph of a left hip.

Reprinted from *Journal of Arthroplasty*, **23**, 8, Spencer, S., Carter, R., Murray, H., and Meek, R.M., 'Femoral neck narrowing after metal-on-metal hip resurfacing', pp. 1105–1109, Copyright 2008, with permission from Elsevier.

What type of bearing is this?

What are its advantages over a conventional bearing surface?

What factors influence the type of lubrication achieved?

Are there any adverse effects with this type of bearing?

What type of bearing is this?

This is a hip resurfacing arthroplasty, with a large-diameter, cobalt–chrome, metal-on-metal bearing.

What are its advantages over a conventional bearing surface?

1. Low wear: after an initial period of bedding-in wear, these devices have a linear wear rate of less than 0.01 mm/year, compared with metal on UHMWPE bearings, which have a linear wear rate of 0.1–0.2 mm/year
2. Hydrodynamic lubrication: hip simulator studies suggest that a large-head metal-on-metal articulation is capable of fluid-film lubrication. It is likely that boundary lubrication occurs when the hip is at rest and a fluid film only when the hip is moving

What factors influence the type of lubrication achieved?

1. Radial clearance: this is the gap between the acetabular and femoral bearing surfaces. A large radial clearance results in polar bearing and boundary lubrication. A small radial clearance may result in equatorial bearing. There is therefore an optimal radial clearance for each size of femoral component, which is small enough to allow fluid-film lubrication but large enough to prevent excessive wear and cold-welding
2. Femoral head diameter: large femoral heads are more likely to induce fluid-film lubrication
3. Component position: a high cup abduction angle can increase the risk of edge loading, which in turn results in boundary lubrication

Are there any adverse effects with this type of bearing?

1. Cancer risk: metal-on-metal articulations produce large numbers of very small wear particles. In addition, high levels of cobalt and chrome are measured in the blood of patients with this type of bearing surface. There is concern, although no definitive evidence, that this may increase the risk of developing some types of cancer
2. Inflammatory masses: some patients with metal-on-metal hip resurfacing arthroplasty have developed large, local inflammatory masses caused by metal wear debris, often requiring revision surgery. Patients in whom these devices were implanted need follow-up according to National Institute for Health and Care Excellence (NICE) guidelines to identify those requiring revision.

Viva 39

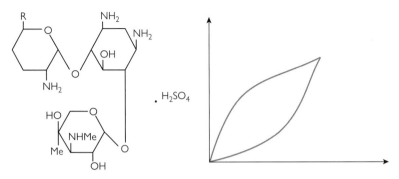

Figure 4.5 A chemical formula of a compound, and a graph illustrating some material properties.

This is the chemical structure of a material we commonly use in joint arthroplasty—what do you think it is?

What is it made of?

Do you know of any changes to cementing techniques over the years?

What happens when the powder and liquid are mixed?

What are its material properties?

What factors influence its properties?

This is the chemical structure of a material we commonly use in joint arthroplasty—what do you think it is?

Bone cement.

What is it made of?

The main components are powder and liquid:

1. Powder:
   - Pre-polymerized poly methyl methacrylate (PMMA)
   - Barium sulphate
2. Liquid:
   - Mono methyl methacrylate (MMA, monomer)
   - N-dimethyl-p-toluidine, which acts as an accelerator
   - Hydroquinone, which acts as an inhibitor
   - Colour, e.g. chlorophyll

Do you know of any changes to cementing techniques over the years?

First generation—hand mixed, no canal preparation, finger packed, no cement restrictor

Second generation—hand mixed, brushed pulsatile lavage, cement gun, inserting the cement retrograde, and distal cement restrictor

Third generation—vacuum mix, brushed pulsatile lavage, cement gun with pressurization and distal canal plug, stem centralizer (can be considered fourth generation)

What happens when the powder and liquid are mixed?

Phase 1. Mixing—add liquid to powder until dough is homogeneous

Phase 2. Waiting—from end of Phase 1 until dough is no longer sticky or hairy

Phase 3. Working—from end of Phase 2 until cement does not join without folds during continuous kneading. At the end of this phase an implant can no longer be inserted

Phase 4. Hardening—during which the cement cures to a hard consistency with a peak in temperature

Phase 2, 3, and 4 are dependent on the ambient temperature. Phase 1 is independent of the temperature.

What are its material properties?

Cement is a viscoelastic material and has the following properties:

1. Creep: increasing strain under a constant load (stress)
2. Stress relaxation: a reduction in stress under a constant strain
3. Hysteresis: refers to the process by which a viscoelastic substance loses energy when a load is applied, then removed

What factors influence its properties?

1. Porosity—vacuum mixing improves fatigue strength
2. Antibiotics

Viva 40

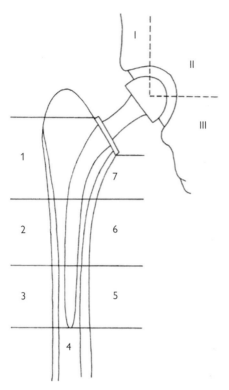

Figure 4.6 Diagrammatical representation of a total hip replacement with labelled zones.

Reproduced from C. Bulstrode et al., *Oxford Textbook of Trauma and Orthopaedics* second edition, 2011, figure 7.10.3, p. 586, with permission from Oxford University Press.

What does this diagram represent?

What is the pathological process behind aseptic loosening?

What does this diagram represent?

The diagram shows the potential areas of lucency around the femoral and acetabular components of a total hip replacement according to Gruen (femur) and DeLee and Charnley (cup).

What is the pathological process behind aseptic loosening?

Osteolysis in total joint replacement is thought to occur as a result of resorption of bone by osteoclasts at the bone–cement interface and is associated with aseptic implant loosening. Polyethylene wear debris produced at the bearing surfaces combined with cement debris formed from movement at the interfaces is thought to induce osteolysis. *In vitro* studies suggest that the activated macrophage is a key intermediary in this process.

Peri-prosthetic bone resorption involves a series of complicated interactions between macrophages and osteoclasts. Osteolysis occurs owing to both the direct resorption of bone, as a consequence of osteoclast stimulation and, to a lesser extent, the secretion of enzymes from other cells (such as metalloproteinases from fibroblasts). Macrophages are thought to be pivotal in the osteolysis process.

Cell culture studies have demonstrated that particulate wear debris from prosthetic materials is *phagocytosed* by macrophages, which subsequently respond in one of two ways:

- First they secrete numerous cellular mediators some of which [tumour necrosis factor-alpha (TNF-α), interleukin (IL)-6, IL-1, and prostaglandin 2 (PGE2)] are able to induce cell proliferation and bone resorption in osteoclasts
- Second, *in vitro* studies have demonstrated that activated macrophages are able to differentiate into osteoclasts via two distinct pathways [fibroblast receptor activator of nuclear factor kappa-B ligand (RANKL) activated and TNF-α activated]

Viva 41

This is a stress–strain curve for a generic material. It represents the material behaviour during a SINGLE loading episode.

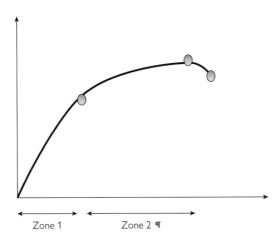

Figure 4.7 A graph of the stress/strain relationship of material.

What does Zone 1 represent?

What is Young's modulus?

What does the first circle represent?

What is Zone 2?

What do the second and third circles represent?

What is strain hardening?

What does Zone 1 represent?

The elastic zone: a material is perfectly elastic if the strain reduces to zero when the stress is removed.

What is Young's modulus?

Young's modulus is stress/strain in the elastic region and is a measure of the stiffness of the material. (The higher the Young's modulus, i.e. steeper the slope, the higher the stiffness.)

What does the first circle represent?

It represents the proportional limit, which is the point at which the zone of elasticity ends. At this point, a sudden elongation of the material occurs without a significant increase in the applied load.

What is Zone 2?

The plastic zone: during this phase the material will not regain its original length when the load is removed.

What do the second and third circles represent?

The second circle is the point of ultimate strength; this is the point of maximum stress. The stress gradually reduces as the strain increases and the material fails at the third circle. The area under the curve represents the 'energy to failure'.

What is strain hardening?

Strain hardening is the increase in stress upon yield stress.

Viva 42

This is a screw from a basic small fragment set used in fracture fixation.

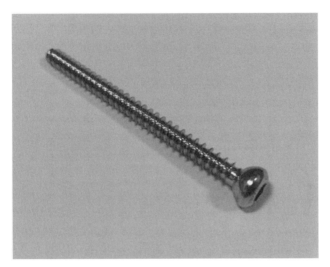

Figure 4.8 Photograph of a surgical screw.
Picture courtesy of Synthes UK Ltd.

Can you take me through the different parts of the screw and their function?

How does the construct of a screw affect its mechanical properties?

How does the small fragment screw differ mechanically from this locking bolt for an intramedullary nail?

What size drills would you use to insert the small fragment screw to act as a lag screw across a fracture?

Can you take me through the different parts of the screw and their function?

Head—provides attachment for a screwdriver (hexagonal for six points of contact to increase torque, avoid slip, and improve directional control).

Counter-sink.

Run out—transitional area between head and thread (relatively weak area).

Shaft—inner core diameter (tensile strength proportional to radius cubed).

Thread—outer diameter (proportional to pull-out strength), partially threaded versus fully threaded (80% grip of near cortex and 20% grip of far cortex).

Crest/root of the thread.

Pitch (lead)—distance advanced for one 360° turn (cancellous > cortical > locking).

Flutes—removes swarf (bone debris).

Tip—difference between cortical (blunt) and cancellous screw (corkscrew).

How does the construct of a screw affect its mechanical properties?

A screw is a device that converts a torsional force into a linear force. Its mechanical properties can be described in terms of its pull-out strength and tensile strength.

The effective thread depth is a combination of pitch and thread (outer diameter), which is proportional to pull-out strength.

The tensile strength is proportional to the inner core radius cubed.

How does the small fragment screw differ mechanically from this locking bolt for an intramedullary nail?

A locking bolt is there to create a rotationally stable construct. It has a wide inner core diameter (ultimate tensile stress, UTS) relative to a small thread (it doesn't need a large amount of pull-out strength).

What size drills would you use to insert the small fragment screw to act as a lag screw across a fracture?

Large lag hole (near cortex) = 3.5 mm drill.

Small hole (far cortex) 2.5 mm.

Chapter 5 Statistics and Orthopaedic Imaging

Viva 43

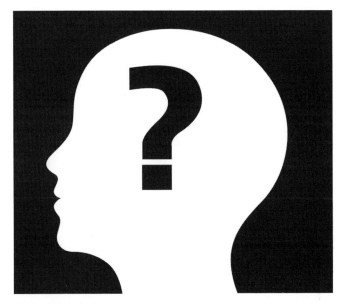

Figure 5.1 A diagram of a head with a question mark.

What is a hypothesis?

What is a null hypothesis?

How would you go about setting up a clinical trial?

What are Type 1 and Type 2 errors?

What is a hypothesis?

A hypothesis is a proposition that serves as a starting point for further investigation.

What is a null hypothesis?

A null hypothesis is a primary assumption that any differences between different groups seen in your study occurred purely by chance.

How would you go about setting up a clinical trial?

1. Identify a problem/interest to be studied—via literature search—and identify a gold standard to compare with
2. Ask a scientific question—define a null hypothesis to test
3. Design your study:
   • Define your population—inclusion/exclusion criteria
   • Methodology of study—randomized/double blinded (masked)/stratification for confounding factors
   • Power analysis (statistician) for numbers required to able to draw statistically valid conclusions from your results
   • Define outcome measures (valid and reproducible)
4. Obtain ethics approval from local or national committee
5. Register trial
6. Conduct the trial
7. Recruit your patients—collect your data
8. Analyse your results (stats)
9. Interpret your findings, write up your work, and publish in peer-reviewed journals

What are Type 1 and Type 2 errors?

A Type 1 or alpha error occurs when a researcher's false hypothesis is accepted—in other words a null hypothesis that is true is falsely rejected or the p-value suggests there is significant difference when there isn't. It is protected against by having high levels of significance. The level that is usually selected for biological studies is 95%.

A Type 2 or beta error occurs when a researcher's hypothesis that is true cannot be demonstrated—in other words a null hypothesis is falsely accepted or the p-value suggests there is no difference when there is. This is protected against by increasing the power of the study, i.e. increasing the numbers being analysed.

Viva 44

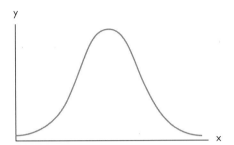

Figure 5.2 A graph illustrating continuous distribution.

What kinds of data are there in orthopaedic surgical literature and what common statistical tests are used for these data?

What do you understand by the sensitivity and specificity of a test?

What factors do you look for in an outcome scoring system?

What kinds of data are there in orthopaedic surgical literature and what common statistical tests are used for these data?

There are discrete data which are also known as non-continuous, qualitative, or categorical (e.g. male or female, Gustilo type 1, 2, 3a, 3b, or 3c). These types of data can be analysed statistically using the chi-squared test or Fisher's exact test.

There are also continuous or variable data, e.g. age, height, erythrocyte sedimentation rate (ESR), knee valgus angle. These data often, but not always, occur in a normal or Gaussian distribution, e.g. a symmetrical bell-shaped curve.

Continuous data can be described using:

- 'Mean', which is the arithmetical average of the data set
- 'Median', which is the middle value of the data set when placed in ascending or descending order
- 'Mode', which is the most frequently occurring value of the data set

In a normal distribution the mean, median, and mode are equal.

'Dispersion' is the variability of a data set. If all the values were the same then the dispersion would be zero. There are various ways of measuring dispersion in statistics including quartiles, standard deviation (SD), and variance. For a set of data the range equals the lowest and highest numbers. The percentiles are groups of data in percentage brackets (usually 25%). The variance is a measure of how much a typical value deviates from the mean (variance = corrected sum of the squares about the mean). The SD is the square root of the variance (to give the same original dimension as the data). In a normal distribution 95% of values are within ±2 SD of the mean. The standard error of the mean (SEM) measures how closely the sample mean of the data set approximates to the population mean that data set was taken from. SEM = SD/$\sqrt{n}$.

Normally distributed data can be compared statistically using parametric statistical tests such as Student's t-test. Data which are not distributed normally require non-parametric tests.

What do you understand by the sensitivity and specificity of a test?

Sensitivity is:

- The ability of a test to detect cases that are positive
- It is equal to (all positive test results/all cases that are truly positive) × 100

Specificity is:

- The ability of a test to detect cases that are negative
- It is equal to (all negative test results/all cases that are truly negative) × 100

What factors do you look for in an outcome scoring system?

Accuracy = how accurate it is compared with a gold standard.

Validity = the extent to which an experimental value represents a true value (the usefulness or utility of a score or test).

Reliability = the ability to repeat the study/test and get the same results.

Ease of use = the assessment method should be appropriate and not too long, complex, or cumbersome.

Viva 45

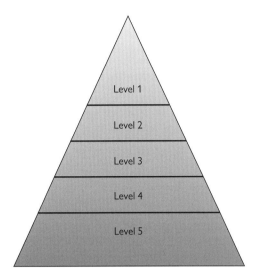

Figure 5.3 A pyramid illustrating types of evidence.

What is a systematic review?

What is a meta-analysis?

What levels of evidence do orthopaedic surgeons recognize?

What types of study do you know about?

What is the difference between bias and confounding?

What is the Cochrane Collaboration?

What is a systematic review?

A systematic review is an overview of primary studies that used explicit and reproducible methods.

What is a meta-analysis?

A meta-analysis is the mathematical and statistical analysis of the combined results of two or more studies that addressed the same hypothesis in the same way.

What levels of evidence do orthopaedic surgeons recognize?

1. High-quality randomized controlled trial (RCT)/systematic review
2. Low-quality RCT/prospective comparative cohort study/systematic review
3. Case–control study/retrospective comparative cohort study/systematic review
4. Case report or case series
5. Expert opinion

What types of study do you know about?

Descriptive studies:

- Case reports
- Correlational studies—studies that use large populations and correlate various factors to the presence of disease states
- Cross-sectional studies—studies that look at a particular group at one moment in time

Analytic studies:

- Studies where hypotheses can be tested, e.g. case–control studies, cohort studies, survival analysis, and interventional studies where a particular intervention is tested. The gold-standard interventional study is the randomized double-blind clinical trial

What is the difference between bias and confounding?

Bias is a conscious or unconscious error in the way that cases are selected or measurements are taken in studies. It is often divided into selection bias and observational bias. Confounding occurs when factors not under study affect the results. The confounding factors may be linked to the factors under study.

What is the Cochrane Collaboration?

An international not-for-profit organization preparing, maintaining, and promoting the accessibility of systematic reviews of the effects of health care.

Viva 46

Item	Scoring categories
During the past four weeks	
1) How would you describe the pain you usually had from your hip?	1 None 2 Very mild 3 Mild 4 Moderate 5 Severe
2) Have you had any trouble with washing and drying yourself (all over) because of your hip?	1 No trouble at all 2 Very little trouble 3 Moderate trouble 4 Extreme difficulty 5 Impossible to do
3) Have you had any trouble getting in and out of a car or using public transport because of your hip? (whichever you tend to use)	1 No trouble at all 2 Very little trouble 3 Moderate trouble 4 Extreme difficulty 5 Impossible to do
3) Have you been able to put on a pair of socks, stockings or tights?	1 Yes, easily 2 With little difficulty 3 With moderate difficulty 4 With extreme difficulty 5 No, impossible
3) Could you do the household shopping on your own?	1 Yes, easily 2 With little difficulty 3 With moderate difficulty 4 With extreme difficulty 5 No, impossible

Figure 5.4 A section of a questionnaire.

The picture above shows part of a questionnaire. What sort of questionnaire is this and when is it used?

What other ways are there of assessing outcome from surgery?

How might outcome measures be used in your practice?

The picture above shows part of a questionnaire, what sort of questionnaire is this and when is it used?

These questions actually come from the Oxford Hip Score, although these details are not as important as recognizing that it represents a patient-reported outcome measure (PROM). They are used for assessment of pre-operative pain and function and post-operative outcome.

What other ways are there of assessing outcome from surgery?

Several types of tool are available to describe outcome after hip surgery such as:

- General morbidity and mortality figures
- Generic quality-of-life questionnaires
- Disease-specific quality-of-life questionnaires
- Joint-specific outcome measures

How might outcome measures be used in your practice?

Outcome measures can be used to evaluate process outcome, including the performance of a surgical unit. They may also be used to evaluate a surgical procedure/prosthesis. The Department of Health now requires all patients undergoing joint replacement to have evaluation using the appropriate 'Oxford Score' to audit patient outcome. PROMs have become powerful tools in both clinical practice and clinical research.

Viva 47

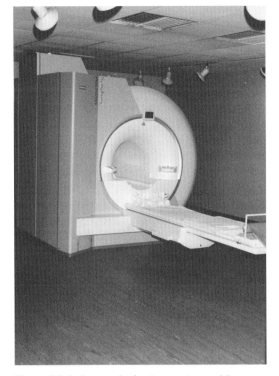

Figure 5.5 A photograph of an investigation modality.

What is this?

What are its component parts?

How does it work?

What is this?

A magnetic resonance imaging (MRI) scanner.

What are its component parts?

It has three main components:

1. A superconducting electromagnet made of a niobium–titanium or niobium–tin alloy and cooled by liquid helium
2. A radiofrequency (RF) system consisting of an RF synthesizer, power amplifier, and transmitting coil
3. Gradient coils: these determine the positions of protons in the scanning field

How does it work?

1. The human body is composed mainly of water, which contains hydrogen nuclei (protons) that spin about their individual axes
2. Protons align with the magnetic field in the MRI scanner and precess in a uniform manner
3. An RF pulse is applied, causing the protons to absorb some of its energy
4. When the RF pulse is removed the protons release their energy as radio waves over different time periods. The term T1 represents the longitudinal relaxation time for the protons while T2 is the relaxation time in the transverse plane
5. The positions of the radio waves are determined by applying pulsed magnetic fields, using the gradient coils

Part 3   **Trauma**

Chapter 6   Lower Limb and Pelvic Trauma

Viva 48

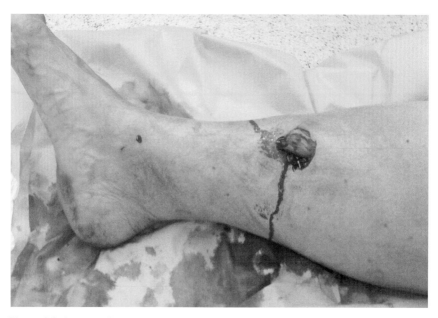

Figure 6.1 A picture of a right lower limb.

This 27 year old has been involved in a road traffic accident (RTA).

Describe what you see in this picture and explain your initial management?

When are you going to take this patient to theatre and what will you plan to do?

What is your biggest concern in the early post-operative period and how do you monitor for this?

How would you perform lower leg fasciotomies?

How soon should you aim to get soft-tissue cover and what do you know about free flaps?

Describe what you see in this picture and explain your initial management?

This is a clinical photograph showing an open fracture of the right tibia. After ruling out more urgent issues with an Advanced Trauma Life Support (ATLS) review, I would assess and document the neurovascular status of the limb, examine the wound, photograph, and then cover with a saline-soaked gauze. I would provide analgesia and splint the limb. I would give intravenous antibiotics and tetanus toxoid, if needed, and obtain antero-posterior (AP) and lateral radiographs.

When are you going to take this patient to theatre and what will you plan to do?

If working at a specialist centre, I would arrange for theatre at the earliest scheduled trauma list (not necessarily < 6 h) according to the British Orthopaedic Association Standards for Trauma and Orthopaedics (BOAST) 4 guideline. Together with a plastic surgeon, I would formulate and document a management plan for both the soft tissues and bone. If working at a non-specialist centre, I would delay surgery and transfer the patient. Urgent surgery is required in some multiply injured patients or if the wound is heavily contaminated with marine, agricultural, or sewage matter.

The optimal surgical result would be skeletal stabilization and wound coverage achieved in a single stage. If this is not possible, then a vacuum foam dressing or an antibiotic bead pouch may be required.

What is your biggest concern in the early post-operative period and how do you monitor for this?

With any high-energy fracture, particularly tibial fractures, I would have a high index of suspicion for compartment syndrome. For this reason, I would avoid regional anaesthetic blocks. In my unit, we monitor patients with regular clinical observation. Invasive pressure monitoring is used for those patients who have a reduced conscious level.

How would you perform lower leg fasciotomies?

I use the two-incision technique as described in the British Orthopaedic Association (BOA)/British Association of Plastic Reconstructive and Aesthetic Surgeons (BAPRAS) guidelines published in 1997. The first longitudinal incision is 1 cm medial to the posteromedial border of the tibia and allows decompression of the posterior compartments. The second incision is placed 2 cm lateral to the anterior border of the tibia and allows access to the anterior and peroneal compartments.

How soon should you aim to get soft-tissue cover and what do you know about free flaps?

The recommendation for definitive soft-tissue cover is within 72 h of initial injury. Soft-tissue coverage may be obtained by delayed primary closure or by one of the techniques of the reconstructive ladder. The most complex of these is the free flap. This usually involves taking a distant muscle with its vascular supply and revascularizing it with healthy vessels close to the recipient site. This muscle is then covered with a split-thickness skin graft.

Viva 49

This patient was the driver in a high-speed RTA.

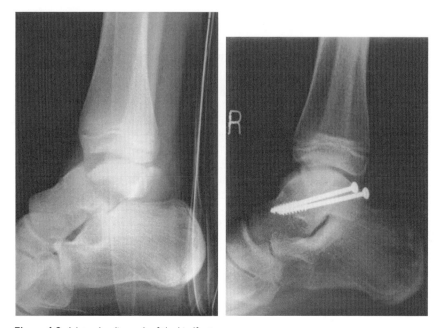

Figure 6.2 A lateral radiograph of the hindfoot.

Reproduced from C. Bulstrode et al., *Oxford Textbook of Trauma and Orthopaedics* second edition, 2011, figure 14.11.3, p. 1717, with permission from Oxford University Press.

What do you see in this picture and what causes this type of injury?

What other information would you like?

What is the standard treatment for this fracture?

What complications should you anticipate in this patient?

What is the probability of AVN in this case and what would you see?

Can you describe the blood supply to the talus?

What do you see in this picture and what causes this type of injury?

This is a lateral radiograph showing a displaced talar neck fracture. The subtalar joint appears to be incongruent.

I would classify this with the Hawkin's system as a type II.

This injury is caused by the application of an axial load to the plantar aspect of the foot. This is a high-energy injury often associated with road traffic collisions.

What other information would you like?

As this is a high-energy fracture I would be concerned about the general status of the patient and whether this was an isolated injury. I would want to have a full ATLS type review. Regarding this injury I would want to know the neurovascular status of the foot and whether it was a closed injury. I would also require further radiographs of the foot/ankle and computerized tomography (CT) scan if available.

What is the standard treatment for this fracture?

Type II and III fractures should be reduced and fixed with two cannulated interfragmentary compression screws. I would use an anteromedial approach to the neck of the talus to openly reduce and fix the fracture from anterior to posterior. My aim would be for anatomical reduction as malunion is associated with poor results.

What complications should you anticipate in this patient?

Early complications include compartment syndrome of the foot. There are a total of nine compartments in the foot. If necessary I would decompress the foot via two dorsal incisions, over the second and fourth metatarsals, and one medial incision. Mid-term complications include: infection, mal/non-union, and avascular necrosis (AVN). Long-term complications include: osteoarthritis.

What is the probability of AVN in this case and what would you see?

AVN risk could be expected to be around 25% in this case. I would expect to see increased density of the talar body followed by subchondral collapse and talar dome fragmentation. I would also look for the Hawkins sign. This is the presence of subchondral lucency seen radiographically around 2 months after fracture. It is a good sign indicating reperfusion of the talus.

Can you describe the blood supply to the talus?

The blood supply to the talus is via an anastomosis formed by three main arteries and their branches. The predominant supply to the talar body is from the posterior tibial via the branch to the tarsal canal. The talar head and neck are supplied by the dorsalis pedis and artery of the sinus tarsi, a branch of the peroneal artery.

Viva 50

This 77-year-old lady fell off her bicycle sustaining this injury.

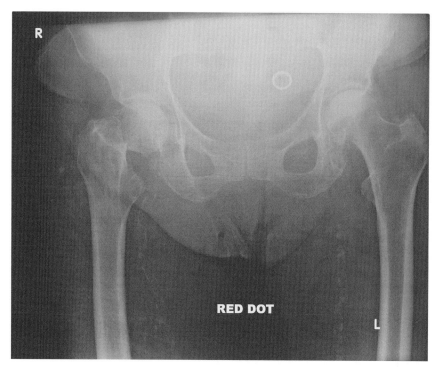

Figure 6.3 An AP pelvis radiograph.

What does this radiograph show and how would you classify this fracture?

What would you like to like to know about the patient?

What is your initial management?

How would you manage this lady?

How would you manage this fracture if it belonged to a 42 year old?

This patient presented at 10 pm—would you operate that night?

What does this radiograph show and how would you classify this fracture?

There is a displaced intracapsular fracture of the right neck of the femur. I would describe this as a Garden IV fracture as there is complete displacement. Clinically the most important classification is simply between displaced and undisplaced fractures.

What would you like to like to know about the patient?

I need to know about any other injuries and the patient's acute medical status. I would then enquire about medical co-morbidities, residential status, and her pre-morbid mobility. Her mental status both acutely and pre-injury are also important.

What is your initial management?

I would manage this patient along the BOAST guidelines. She requires analgesia, plain radiographs, and admission to an appropriate ward within 4 h. Routine bloods and electrocardiogram (ECG) are performed and the patient rehydrated. I would plan for surgery within 48 h unless a reversible medical condition was present.

How would you manage this lady?

After following the guidelines as previously described, I would discuss treatment with this lady and propose a total hip replacement (THR). Studies show that patients do better functionally with a THR and re-operation rates are lower. I would certainly expect this particular lady to do better with a THR. I would use a cemented cup and stem with a 32-mm head via a modified Hardinge approach.

I would have a multidisciplinary approach to her management, including input from an orthogeriatrician and daily physiotherapy.

How would you manage this fracture if it belonged to a 42 year old?

I would aim to conserve the femoral head by reducing the fracture under direct visualization and fixing internally with three cannulated screws.

This patient presented at 10 pm—would you operate that night?

I would operate the next morning as evidence suggests that rapid surgery does not affect outcome. The most important factor is accurate reduction.

Viva 51

This rugby player landed awkwardly after a lineout.

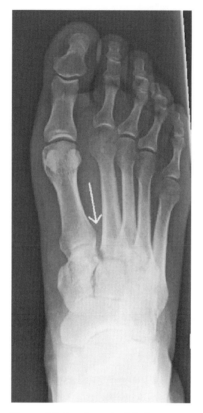

Figure 6.4 A radiograph of the foot.

Reproduced from Aneel Bhangu, Caroline Lee, and Keith Porter, *Emergencies in Trauma*, 2010, figure 11.13, p. 198, with permission from Oxford University Press.

What do you see and which joint is involved?

What is the Lisfranc joint?

How do you describe Lisfranc injuries and which type is this?

This is an isolated injury, how would you proceed?

What do you look for on plain radiographs?

What is your operative plan for this fracture?

What are you going to say to this patient about his long-term outcome?

What do you see and which joint is involved?

This AP radiograph shows disruption at the tarso-metatarsal joints, otherwise known as a Lisfranc injury. There is a fracture through the base of the second metatarsal with displacement of several of the lesser metatarsals. The hallux metatarsal appears to be undisplaced.

What is the Lisfranc joint?

This consists of three cuneiform and two cuboid metatarsal articulations. Joint stability is provided by strong ligaments and the recessing of the second metatarsal base. The Lisfranc ligament runs from the base of the second metatarsal to the medial cuneiform.

How do you describe Lisfranc injuries and which type is this?

Type A is a complete uniplanar dislocation involving the whole joint. A type B injury describes a partial dislocation, either medial or lateral. Type C injuries are divergent dislocations. In this case there appears to be a lateral type B injury.

This is an isolated injury, how would you proceed?

I would provide analgesia and elevation with a resting splint, including the foot and ankle, but allowing room for swelling. I would observe for evidence of compartment syndrome and obtain further radiographic views and CT scan. I would wait for the swelling to reduce before considering surgery. Skin softening and wrinkling suggests that swelling is receding.

What do you look for on plain radiographs?

On an AP view the second metatarsal and medial cuneiform medial borders should align. On an oblique view the medial borders of the fourth metatarsal and cuboid should align. I would also look for the fleck sign, which implies an avulsion of the Lisfranc ligament.

What is your operative plan for this fracture?

I would plan to openly reduce and fix with screws, starting with the second metatarsal reduction. I would employ two skin incisions, one in line with the first web space, the second over the fourth metatarsal. Sometimes a smaller incision is required for introduction of a Lisfranc screw (cuboid to bone of second metatarsal)

What are you going to say to this patient about his long-term outcome?

I would warn him that even if his surgery goes well and things heal as planned there remains a 30% chance of post-traumatic osteoarthritis.

Viva 52

This 40 year old sustained this injury in a high-speed car collision.

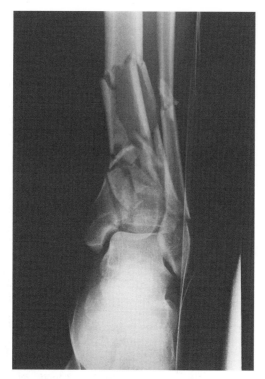

Figure 6.5 AP radiograph of the left ankle.

Reproduced from C. Bulstrode et al., *Oxford Textbook of Trauma and Orthopaedics* second edition, 2011, figure 12.15.4, p. 973, with permission from Oxford University Press.

Describe what you see in this picture and explain your initial management?

What is your primary treatment upon admission?

Do you know a way of classifying these fractures?

How would you definitively treat this fracture?

What are the AO principles?

What complications are you going to warn the patient about?

Describe what you see in this picture and explain your initial management?

This is an AP and lateral radiograph centred on the left ankle. There is a multifragmentary pilon fracture and transverse fracture of the fibula. I would perform an ATLS review and rule out concomitant injuries. I would then assess the neurovascular status of the affected limb and observe for signs of open injury or degloving. I would apply a temporary splint, provide analgesia, and obtain repeat AP and lateral radiographs.

What is your primary treatment upon admission?

I would plan to take the patient to theatre and place a spanning external fixator. This would keep the limb out to length, maintain alignment, and most importantly avoid further insult to the soft tissues. I would also commence monitoring for signs of compartment syndrome.

Do you know a way of classifying these fractures?

The Rüedi, Matter, and Allgöwer (1979)[1] system describes three fracture types. Type 1 are essentially undisplaced; type 2 are displaced with little fragmentation; and type 3 fractures, like this one, have metaphyseal or articular fragmentation.

How would you definitively treat this fracture?

I would obtain a CT scan to enable pre-op planning. I would consider discussing this patient with a specialist trauma centre. I would expect to wait around 7–10 days for the soft tissues to be in an appropriate condition for surgery. I would plan to openly reduce and fix along AO principles paying careful attention to the soft tissues. Non-surgical treatment is an option but would give poor results in this case. Definitive external fixation would be a possibility, such as a fine-wire Ilizarov type frame.

What are the AO principles?

To appropriately restore bony anatomy, to maintain reduction while also respecting soft tissues, and to provide an environment that allows healing and early joint mobilization.

What complications are you going to warn the patient about?

I would discuss short-term complications such as wound breakdown/infection, and compartment syndrome, and also a long-term limitation of ankle movements. I would warn that there is an 80% chance of developing post-traumatic osteoarthritis, although the symptoms from this may be variable.

[1] T. Rüedi, P. Matter, M. Allgöwer. Intra-articular fractures of the distal tibial end. Helv Chir Acta 1968 Nov;35(5):556-82. PMID: 4974693.

Viva 53

This 26-year-old skier crashed.

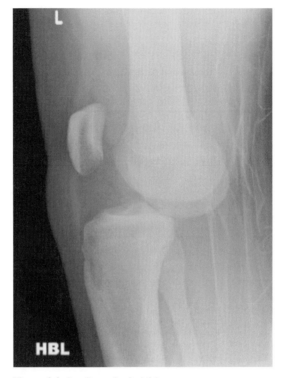

Figure 6.6 A radiograph of a left knee.

What does this radiograph tell you and what are your immediate concerns about the patient?

How do you carry out an initial assessment of this patient?

How do you classify these injuries?

This patient has an arterial injury, how will you proceed?

Which nerve is most commonly damaged and how would you manage this?

How do you provide definitive treatment for an unstable knee?

What does this radiograph tell you and what are your immediate concerns about the patient?

This radiograph shows a rotatory dislocation of the left knee. This is usually a high-energy injury so I would be concerned about general patient status and other injuries. As far as this injury is concerned I would be most worried about a popliteal artery injury, which occurs in around 25% of patients with this injury.

How do you carry out an initial assessment of this patient?

I would assess and document the neurovascular status of the limb before reducing this dislocation, under sedation, as an emergency. After reduction I would again perform a careful neurovascular examination. If there is any suggestion of vascular injury, exploration or angiography is indicated. A 'normal' pulse may not exclude injury; an ankle-brachial pressure index of < 0.9 is abnormal.

How do you classify these injuries?

These injuries are classified according to the direction of dislocation of the tibia in relation to the femur. Anterior dislocations are most common followed by posterior, lateral, medial, and rotatory dislocations. Up to 20% of knee dislocations have spontaneously relocated and do not, therefore, fit into this classification. An alternative way of classifying is by description of ligamentous damage incurred.

This patient has an arterial injury, how will you proceed?

I would arrange for this patient to go urgently to a theatre where a plastic or vascular surgeon will be available. Prompt reconstruction takes priority and would normally involve an interpositional vein graft. The knee would be stabilized, and thus the repair protected, by placing a spanning external fixator. Lower limb fasciotomies are also performed to avoid a reperfusion compartment syndrome.

Which nerve is most commonly damaged and how would you manage this?

The common peroneal nerve is the most frequently involved occurring in around 20–30% of cases. I would treat this expectantly, although a large proportion will not fully recover.

How do you provide definitive treatment for an unstable knee?

I would obtain a magnetic resonance imaging (MRI) scan to characterize ligamentous structures that have been damaged. Associated fractures must also be sought. Additional information may be found by performing an examination under anaesthetic. Repair and/or reconstruction of ligamentous structures should be performed by somebody with experience in this area. Treatment choices lie between early reconstruction of posterolateral corner (PLC) and posterior cruciate ligament (PCL), with delayed anterior cruciate ligament (ACL) reconstruction, and early bracing/rehabilitation with late reconstruction.

Viva 54

This patient was the passenger in a high-speed car crash.

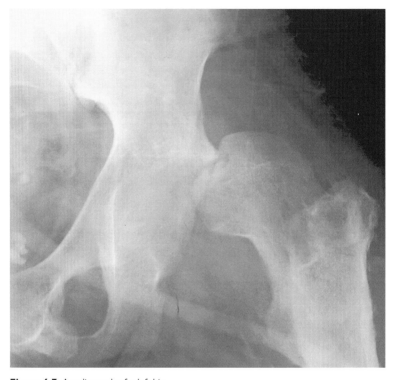

Figure 6.7 A radiograph of a left hip.

Reproduced from C. Bulstrode et al., *Oxford Textbook of Trauma and Orthopaedics* second edition, 2011, figure 12.50.17, p. 1308, with permission from Oxford University Press.

What does this radiograph show you and what would your initial management in the emergency department be?

Once in theatre how would you plan to treat this injury?

What would your management be once you have reduced the dislocation?

What are the indications for fixing the posterior wall fracture?

How would you fix this fracture and what complications would you warn the patient about?

What does this radiograph show you and what would your initial management in the emergency department be?

This is an AP radiograph of the right hip showing a posterior dislocation. There is an associated fracture of the posterior wall of the acetabulum. The femoral head and neck appear to be intact. This is a high-energy injury and with a high probability of other injuries. I would therefore perform a full ATLS type review. I would assess and document the neurovascular status of the limb and provide adequate analgesia. I would liaise with theatres and seek the advice from my local pelvic specialist centre.

Once in theatre how would you plan to treat this injury?

I would initially attempt a closed reduction of the hip. This is done using Bigelow's manoeuvre. With the patient supine and an assistant fixing the pelvis via the anterior superior iliac spines, the surgeon applies traction, adducts, and internally rotates the femur. The majority of dislocations will reduce with this manoeuvre. If the dislocation won't reduce then an emergency open reduction is indicated via a posterior approach.

What would your management be once you have reduced the dislocation?

I would confirm reduction on table with an image intensifier and perform an examination under anaesthetic (EUA) to assess stability. I would place a distal femoral pin for traction to maintain hip reduction. Post-operatively I would request further radiographic imaging including a CT scan. This would confirm concentric reduction, rule out fragments within the joint, and characterize the posterior wall acetabular fracture. When the patient has recovered from the anaesthetic I would repeat my neurovascular examination.

What are the indications for fixing the posterior wall fracture?

The indications for surgery are a lack of joint congruity or instability. Usually if only around 20% of the wall is affected the joint will be stable. Those with between 20 and 40% affected may or may not be unstable. In a young patient such as this, any greater involvement than 30% would be an indication for surgery.

How would you fix this fracture and what complications would you warn the patient about?

I would use a posterior or Kocher-Langenbeck approach for this fracture. Screw fixation alone will be inadequate to maintain reduction and buttress plating will be required. I would warn the patient about early complications such as infection and sciatic nerve damage. Longer-term complications include: heterotopic ossification (HO), AVN, and osteoarthritis. We routinely give indomethacin to reduce the risk of HO and give low-molecular-weight heparin to reduce the risk of deep vein thrombosis and pulmonary embolus.

Viva 55

This 32-year-old pedestrian was hit by a car.

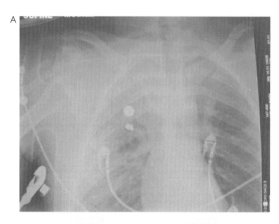

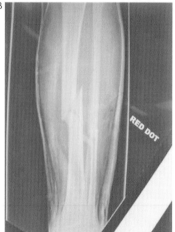

Figure 6.8 An AP radiograph of a right lower limb, and a chest X-ray.

What do you see in these two radiographs?

What do you understand by the term damage control orthopaedics (DCO)?

How do you decide which patients require DCO and what is the alternative?

What is the ISS?

When do you expect to operate definitively on a DCO patient?

What do you see in these two radiographs?

There is an AP view of the tibia that shows a segmental fracture probably resulting from a high-energy impact. The chest radiograph suggests that there has been a significant insult to the chest/lungs.

What do you understand by the term damage control orthopaedics (DCO)?

DCO is a planned and staged surgical strategy in the management of polytrauma patients to minimize the effects of the 'second hit' on an already limited physiological reserve. The 'first hit' is from the injury and the body's response to this injury, while the 'second hit' is produced by surgical intervention. Evidence shows that in certain patients, primary external fixation of long bone fractures and secondary nailing improves outcome. There is a reduction in the incidence of multiple organ dysfunction syndrome (MODS) and adult respiratory distress syndrome (ARDS).

How do you decide which patients require DCO and what is the alternative?

The alternative way of managing polytrauma patients is known as early total care. This preceded the concept of DCO and involves the early treatment of all fractures. Patients who would be suitable for DCO include: those with an injury severity score (ISS) > 20 with chest injury, those with abdominal or pelvic trauma in hypovolaemic shock (SBP < 90mmHg), and anyone with bilateral lung contusions.

What is the ISS?

This is a scoring system based on the abbreviated injury scale (AIS). Each body system is given an AIS of 1–6, with 6 being the most serious. The ISS is calculated by adding the squares of the three most severely injured body systems. A patient with a score > 16 is defined as being seriously injured. In this case a patient has a > 10% risk of mortality.

When do you expect to operate definitively on a DCO patient?

This decision will be made in conjunction with the anaesthetist and intensivist. I would usually expect this to be after at least 4 days. Parameters such as blood pressure, heart rate, arterial blood gases, and core temperature must be corrected to avoid the risk of a large second hit. I would want to exchange from external fixator to a nail within 10 days to avoid an increased infection risk.

Viva 56

This 20-year-old roofer fell from his ladder sustaining this isolated injury.

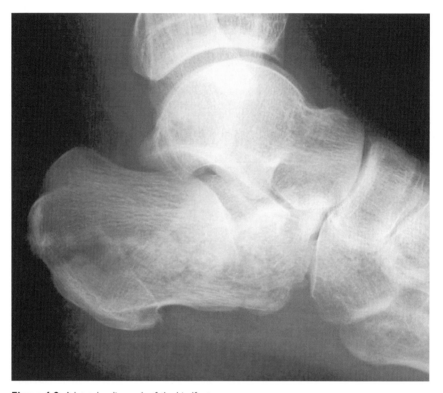

Figure 6.9 A lateral radiograph of the hindfoot.

Reproduced from C. Bulstrode et al., *Oxford Textbook of Trauma and Orthopaedics* second edition, 2011, figure 12.61.9, p. 1419, with permission from Oxford University Press.

What do you see in this radiograph?

What is your management of this patient in the emergency department?

Which further investigations would you order and how are these helpful?

How would you best treat this fracture?

Are you familiar with any published evidence in this area?

What do you see in this radiograph?

This lateral hindfoot radiograph shows a fragmented calcaneal fracture with involvement of the subtalar joint. Bohler's and Gissane's angles are both reduced. Bohler's angle is normally between 20° and 40°; a reduction in this angle implies involvement of the posterior facet.

What is your management of this patient in the emergency department?

I would perform an ATLS review and look for associated injuries. More specifically I would assess the soft tissues and look for open wounds. I would assess and document the neurovascular status of the foot. I would then provide elevation and analgesia before obtaining plain radiographs of the calcaneum and foot. Clinical monitoring for signs of compartment syndrome would be commenced.

Which further investigations would you order and how are these helpful?

I would like further radiographic views including Broden's views, which help to visualize the anterior surface of the posterior facet. I would also request an AP view of the foot to assess the calcaneocuboid joint. I would also request a CT scan. This provides a better understanding of the fracture configuration. CT also allows classification as described by Sanders. The Sanders classification of calcaneal fractures is based upon the position of the primary fracture line and the number of secondary fragments in the posterior facet.

How would you best treat this fracture?

The best treatment continues to be contentious. I believe that with good anatomical reduction, especially of the subtalar joint, the outcome will be improved. I would also discuss non-operative options and emphasize the potential risks of surgery. I would warn the patient that he is unlikely ever to have a 'normal' foot and that his career may well be affected.

Are you familiar with any published evidence in this area?

In 2002, Buckley et al. published a prospective, multi-centre, randomized controlled trial in the *Journal of Bone and Joint Surgery* (American volume), which identified certain subgroups expected to have better or worse surgical outcomes. They studied over 400 patients with displaced intra-articular calcaneal fractures. Around 75% of these were followed up at between 2 and 8 years. Overall the outcomes after non-operative treatment were not found to be different from those after operative treatment. Those patients, however, who were younger, female, or had an anatomical reduction, scored significantly higher on the scoring scales after surgery compared with those who were treated non-operatively.

Viva 57

This lady fell while out shopping.

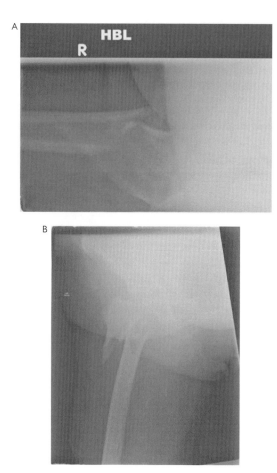

Figure 6.10 An AP and lateral radiograph of the right hip.

What can you tell me about this radiograph?

Who gets subtrochanteric fractures and how do you classify them?

How would you manage this patient in the pre-operative phase?

How do you fix these fractures?

When do you expect union and what is the risk of non-union?

What can you tell me about this radiograph?

This lady has had a previous injury on the right side treated with a sliding hip screw. On the left side there is a displaced subtrochanteric fracture. There is no evidence that this is a pathological fracture. Often in these fractures the proximal fragment lies flexed and in varus owing to the unopposed pull of the iliopsoas. In this case the lesser trochanter has remained with the distal fragment so this deformity would not be seen.

Who gets subtrochanteric fractures and how do you classify them?

This is predominantly a fracture of the elderly. Although relatively uncommon, incidence is rising. Most are caused by simple falls from standing height. A significant portion of these fractures are pathological in origin. In young patients this fracture would invariably be due to a high-energy injury. A universally accepted fracture classification does not exist. Classification is difficult because of different definitions of what constitutes a subtrochanteric fracture. The Russell–Taylor classification divides fractures into four types. This classification describes piriform fossa involvement and medial buttress stability and acts as a guide to reconstruction.

How would you manage this patient in the pre-operative phase?

I would initially assess the patients' acute medical condition and exclude other injuries. I would then check neurovascular status, provide analgesia, and immobilize the limb with a Thomas splint. I would obtain further radiographs including the whole femur. A thorough medical history is required as the association with metastatic disease is high.

How do you fix these fractures?

Historically these fractures were plated, with nailing being a more recent option. All fixation methods have a sizeable failure rate, which makes this a challenging area. The underlying problem is the massive biomechanical loads transmitted through this area. For this particular fracture I would use a cephalomedullary nail.

When do you expect union and what is the risk of non-union?

I would expect union to take around 4 months. This is a classic case of the race between fracture union and implant failure owing to fatigue. Non-union risk would be in the region of 5–10%.

Viva 58

A 35-year-old man is brought to the A&E having been involved in a motorcycle crash at high speed.

A   B

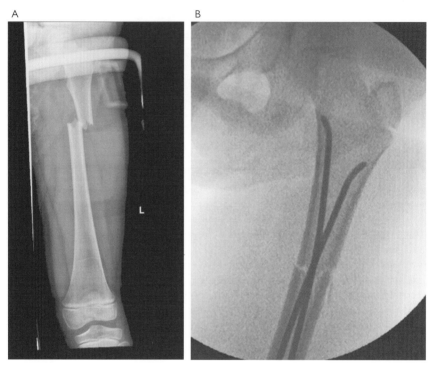

Figure 6.11 An AP pelvis radiograph.

Reproduced from Mihra S. Taljanovic et al., *Musculoskeletal Imaging* Volume 1, 2019, figure 18.6, p. 90, with permission from Oxford University Press.

Describe the radiograph.

How would you manage him initially and definitively?

Describe the radiograph

This is an AP radiograph of the pelvis showing an open-book injury with massive disruption of the sacroiliac joint on the left side. There is also an acetabular fracture on the right side. This would indicate a high-energy injury with significant increased risk of associated injuries.

How would you manage him initially and definitively?

I would manage this patient with the help of a multidisciplinary trauma team following ATLS and BOAST 3 guidelines. Starting with the primary survey, with simultaneous assessment and treatment of any airway, breathing, or circulation problems. The C spine should be immobilized with collar, sandbags, and tape. With the anaesthetist looking after airway and breathing I would concentrate on C because this injury is associated with significant blood loss into the pelvic space. He would require immediate IV access (×2 14 G cannulae placed in the antecubital fossa (ACF)—and bloods sent off for cross-match six units of blood. I would give a fluid challenge of 2 l of warmed Hartmann's. If available I would apply a pelvic binder to close his pubic symphysis diastasis. If not readily available a simpler manoeuvre would be to use a white linen sheet around the pelvis, as well as internally rotating his legs and tying his ankles together. He would require an abdominal assessment by the general surgeons [with a focused assessment with sonography in trauma (FAST) scan] including per rectal (PR) and per vaginal (PV) (beware of occult open fractures). There is a significant chance of a urethral injury in this case and I wouldn't catheterize the patient without a formal review from the urological surgeons.

This is a highly unstable injury pattern. I would take advice from my local pelvic trauma centre. Regarding the application of a temporary external fixator, I would apply this in theatre under a general anaesthetic. Having defined the surface anatomy, I would make small stab incisions over the anterior superior iliac spine (ASIS), and use free-hand k wires either side of the iliac crest in order to place fixator pins in the middle of the bone. I would reduce the diastasis and hold with a cross bar (low down to allow the necessary access needed by general surgeons for laparotomy).

Principles of definitive fixation of this injury can be divided into treating the diastasis, the posterior disruption, and the acetabulum. If the symphysis disruption was well reduced, the fixator could be used definitively. Alternatively, it could be removed and the diastasis held reduced with two reconstructive plates at 90° (this improves stability of the construct). For the sacroiliac (SI) joint disruption, the options include: open reduction internal fixation (ORIF) via a posterior approach and fixation with SI rods or specialized plates, or percutaneous SI joint screw fixation using Flouroscopic (II) control. The management of the acetabular fracture would require three-dimensional CT planning and input from a specialist pelvic trauma unit.

Viva 59

This 5-year-old boy fell out of a tree sustaining a closed isolated injury to his right thigh.

A

B

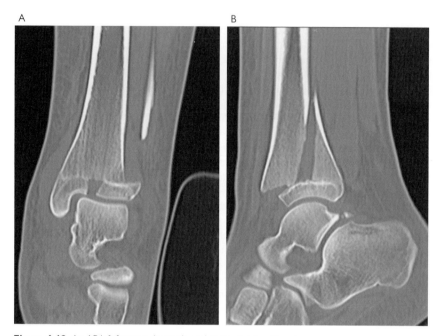

Figure 6.12 An AP left femur radiograph, and an image intensifier view.

What do you see on his X-rays?

What is this fixation? Are you familiar with it?

What are its advantages and disadvantages?

What do you see on his X-rays?

A transverse fracture of the left femoral diaphysis in an immature skeleton. The proximal femur has been flexed and abducted under the forces of iliopsoas and the abductors. The fracture has been splinted with a Thomas splint.

One should be wary of non-accidental injury in a non-walking child.

What is this fixation? Are you familiar with it?

The fracture has been internally fixed with two elastic nails. These have been introduced from a retrograde position, proximal to the physis. It is a good but technically demanding technique that allows for percutaneous entry and minimal soft-tissue trauma. The nails should not exceed a diameter of one-third of the diameter of the medullary canal. Both nails should be the same diameter, to prevent uneven forces, and should be pre-bent before insertion. It relies upon three-point fixation for stability. A retrograde technique is used for midshaft and proximal third fractures. Newer type nails have end caps that screw into the end and prevent backing out—easier to find and remove.

What are its advantages and disadvantages?

Advantages include: minimally invasive technique/triplane stability/rapid healing with callus/no damage to growth plates

Disadvantages include: technically demanding/tip irritation/leg-length discrepancy (LLD) and overgrowth therefore need to be followed carefully.

Viva 60

This 13-year-old boy twisted his ankle falling off his skateboard.

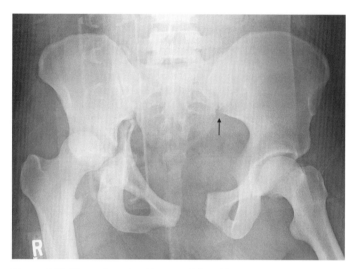

Figure 6.13 Three-dimensional imaging of the ankle.

Can you comment on the imaging?

Why do this age group get these types of fracture pattern?

How would you manage this patient now?

How does this fracture differ from a Tillaux fracture?

Can you comment on the imaging?

The CT slices show coronal and sagittal cuts through the ankle joint. They show a displaced triplane injury typical of an adolescent near skeletal maturity. The sagittal cut shows a Salter–Harris II type appearance and the coronal cut shows a Salter–Harris III type.

Why do this age group get these types of fracture pattern?

The distal tibial physis fuses in a set pattern, starting centrally then medially and finally laterally, which in this age group results in relative weaker areas susceptible to an external rotation torsional force. There are usually two main fragments but sometimes there are three so a CT scan is useful to assess the degree of fragmentation and displacement of the articular surface.

How would you manage this patient now?

The principles of management are to treat the soft tissues and to achieve articular congruity. If this cannot be achieved closed, with internal rotation, then open reduction and internal fixation will be necessary. Small cannulated, partially threaded screws are utilized to stabilize the articular surface and the physis. The patient is then placed in a cast and kept non-weight bearing until callus is present.

How does this fracture differ from a Tillaux fracture?

A Tillaux fracture is an avulsion injury secondary to an external rotation force. It is a Salter–Harris III injury and comes about as the antero-lateral aspect of the distal tibial physis is last to close, and hence fails with the external rotation force. Closed reduction can occasionally be achieved with internal rotation. Open reduction is usually required to remove trapped periosteum, allowing exact reduction, followed by internal fixation with partially threaded cannulated screws. Six weeks in plaster is then required.

Chapter 7 Spine and Upper Extremity Trauma

Viva 61

A 35-year-old man has been involved in a motocross accident and fallen off his bike. Wearing all the protective clothing and helmet he is brought into the emergency department complaining of neck pain.

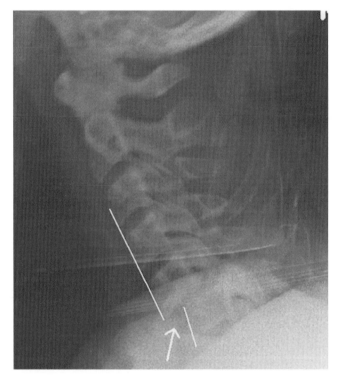

Figure 7.1 C spine radiographs

Reproduced from Aneel Bhangu, Caroline Lee, and Keith Porter, *Emergencies in Trauma*, 2010, figure 13.1, p. 268, with permission from Oxford University Press.

What are your comments about the radiograph?

How would you manage him now?

You don't have access to a magnetic resonance imaging (MRI) scanner, could you reduce this with the patient awake?

How would you apply a Halo?

What are your comments about this radiograph?

He has a step at C5/C6 that is greater than 50% of the vertebral body width, and the facet joints have dislocated. Such an appearance is associated with a bifacetal facet dislocation. The radiograph only shows down to C7 and is therefore inadequate for a trauma C spine lateral radiograph.

How would you manage him now?

I would manage this patient according to Advanced Trauma Life Support (ATLS) guidelines. I would initially remove the helmet visor to gain access to the eyes, nose, and mouth. I would then remove his protective equipment while maintaining spinal immobilization. One needs to exclude other spinal injuries, and obtain full imaging of the spine. Having carried out a full neurological examination, and ensured that this is an isolated injury, I would then contact a specialist spinal surgeon for advice on reduction. This can be a closed awake or open, general anaesthetic (GA) reduction. It is important to exclude a prolapsed disc, which may damage the cord during reduction.

You don't have access to a magnetic resonance imaging (MRI) scanner, could you reduce this with the patient awake?

Yes you can, as long as the patient is awake, alert, and serial neurological examinations are possible. This is controversial. It is carried out by applying Gardner–Wells tongs to the skull and then adding sequential weights to the traction cord. The patient is supine, and an image intensifier is used to image the spine after each additional load is added. Ten pounds is added initially, and then approximately 5 lb per level. Once the neck is fully stretched and the facets have been unlocked, the neck is then extended to complete the reduction, and the traction reduced.

How would you apply a Halo?

I would explain to the patient how and why I am going to do it. Four pins are used after local anaesthetic to the scalp, tightened with a torque limiter (six for a child).
Placement is essential for:

1. Stability of construct—equidistant and symmetrical
2. To prevent damage to important structures—temporal artery/supraorbital nerves/sinuses
   - Anterior—1 cm above lateral outer third eyebrow, eyes closed
   - Posterior—behind earlobe above mastoid

Procedure:

Three-person job—one holding head/two applying
Apply jacket—appropriately sized
Check radiograph of the spine to ensure correct reduction maintained
Tighten the pins after 24 h

Complications:

Loss reduction/position
Pin site infection
Pin loosening
Pain
Nerve injury

Viva 62

This 35-year-old left-handed gentleman sustained this injury while arm wrestling.

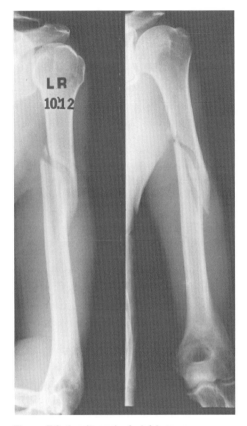

Figure 7.2 A radiograph of a left humerus

Reproduced from C. Bulstrode et al., *Oxford Textbook of Trauma and Orthopaedics* second edition, 2011, figure 12.11.8, p. 937, with permission from Oxford University Press.

Describe the radiograph to me. How would you go about managing this injury?

It's documented by the casualty officer that he has a dense radial nerve palsy. How would this alter your management?

You've managed his radial nerve palsy expectantly but after 4 months there has been no improvement. What would you do now?

What are the principles of tendon transfers? Which would you use here?

Describe the radiograph to me. How would you go about managing this injury?

This is an oblique radiograph of the left humerus showing a spiral fracture of the distal diaphysis. I would like to see another view, making sure this was an isolated injury. I would give the patient some analgesia and a collar and cuff sling. I would take a mechanism of injury history and then examine the arm assessing the soft tissues (open?/compartment syndrome?) and distal neurovascular status (particularly radial pulse and radial nerve function). I would then take a more detailed general history—personality of patient.

You could treat this non-operatively with analgesia and gravity traction in collar and cuff; however, I would have a low threshold for fixation in distal third fractures, which are prone to slip into varus. For operative fixation I would use a posterior approach:

- Position—patient on their side and the arm over a well-padded roll
- Approach—using a midline skin incision the plane is between the lateral and long head triceps—which is easier to find proximally (no true internervous plane—but muscles innervated very high up so are not denervated). I would look for the radial nerve and profunda artery in the spiral groove coming medial to lateral—find and protect. I would then split the medial head in line of fibres on to the bone (subperiosteal). More distally, beware the ulna nerve as it comes from the anterior compartment to the posterior compartment distally on the medial side
- Reduction and fixation—I would use a lag screw (large fragment set) and then a 4.5-mm broad dynamic compression plate (DCP) with four bicortical screws on each side (screws are offset)
- Op note—I would document the position of the nerve in relation to the plate.

It's documented by the casualty officer that he has a dense radial nerve palsy. How would this alter your management?

Treat the radial nerve injury expectantly (90% are neuropraxias and recover within 3–4 months). Provide a wrist splint (in extension) for wrist drop/physio to maintain passive range of movement.

You've managed his radial nerve palsy expectantly but after 4 months there has been no improvement. What would you do now?

I would organize nerve conduction and electromyography (EMG) studies. If these showed a neuropraxia, I would continue to monitor expectantly. If the muscle is denervated (axon or neurotemesis), the muscle will show fibrillation potentials on EMGs (secondary to a hypersensitive post-synaptic membrane and random release of pockets of Ach). I would refer to the local peripheral nerve injury specialist unit (after waiting at least 6 months from injury).

What are the principles of tendon transfers? Which would you use here?

Tendon transfer is the late option, the principles of which are:

- A supple joint with full range of passive motion
- Healthy donor that is expendable with grade 5 Medical Research Council (MRC) power (lose one grade with transfer), adequate excursion, with a synergist with a straight line of pull
- Good recipient site—tendon of paralysed muscle (if this is the reason for transfer)
- For a high radial nerve palsy, common transfers include: pronator teres to extensor carpi radialis brevis (ECRB), palmaris longus to extensor pollicis longus (EPL), and flexor carpi radialis (FCR) to extensor digitorum (ED)

Viva 63

A 25-year-old man is brought into casualty with a closed isolated injury of his non-dominant left arm.

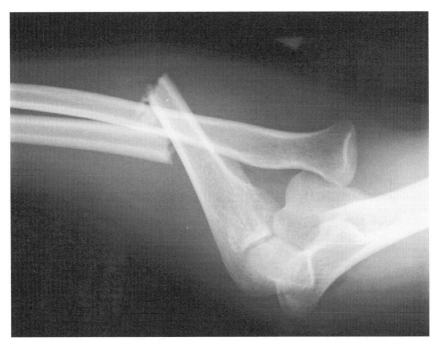

Figure 7.3 A radiograph of an elbow

Reproduced from Aneel Bhangu, Caroline Lee, and Keith Porter, *Emergencies in Trauma*, 2010, figure 12.12, p. 234, with permission from Oxford University Press.

Can you describe the injury to me?

How do you classify these injuries?

How would you manage this patient?

You choose to open and reduce the ulna fracture under direct vision and fix it with a DCP. Tell me how this plate works.

Can you describe the injury to me?

This is an antero-posterior (AP) radiograph of the left elbow showing a Monteggia fracture dislocation. I would like to see further views of the whole forearm as well as a lateral view of the elbow to determine the exact direction of dislocation of the radial head.

How do you classify these injuries?

Classification of Monteggia fractures uses the Bado system and is determined by the direction of radial head dislocation:

1. Anterior (60)%
2. Posterior (15%—more common in adults than children)
3. Lateral (15–25%)
4. Any: with associated radial shaft fracture (rare)

How would you manage this patient?

Management of this isolated injury can be divided into initial A&E management and definitive management. I would first assess the patient in A&E giving some analgesia and taking a full history. On examination I would check the soft tissues for any evidence of open fracture or compartment syndrome as well as documenting carefully the distal neurovascular status. The posterior interosseus nerve is particularly at risk. This fracture dislocation needs to be reduced and fixed urgently. I would organize for the patient to go to theatre when medically safe. In theatre I would use a direct approach to the ulna shaft utilizing the internervous plane between the extensor carpi ulnaris (ECU) (posterior interosseous nerve, PIN) and flexor carpi ulnaris (FCU) (ulnar nerve, UN). I would reduce the fracture under direct vision and then check whether the radial head had relocated with image intensifier. I would fix this fracture with a 3.5-mm DCP using AO principles.

You choose to open and reduce the ulna fracture under direct vision and fix it with a DCP. Tell me how this plate works

Compression can be applied across the fracture in a number of different ways. First, by pre-bending the plate; second, by placing the screws eccentrically in the combihole to allow sliding compression at the fracture site; and, third, by utilizing the compression device via a separately placed screw adjacent to the plate.

Post-operatively, I would protect the soft tissues in a backslab for 4 weeks to prevent late subluxation of radial head. The patient would then require physiotherapy to regain elbow motion.

Viva 64

A 19-year-old rugby player presents to A&E with a first -time injury to his dominant shoulder.

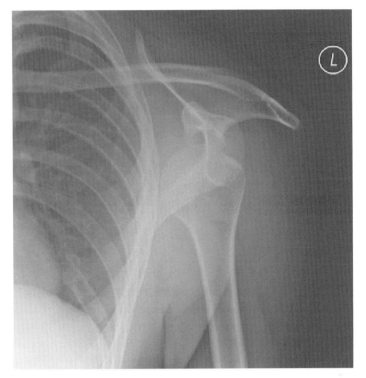

Figure 7.4 A radiograph of a left shoulder

Reproduced from Philip G. Conaghan, Philip O'Connor, and David A. Isenberg, *Oxford Specialist Handbook: Musculoskeletal Imaging*, figure 4.6, p. 105, 2010, with permission from Oxford University Press.

Comment on the radiograph.

Why does the shoulder dislocate? What stops it normally?

The A&E staff have tried to reduce this without success—talk me through how you would reduce this dislocation.

What is the risk of this shoulder causing problems again?

What approach would you take for an open reduction?

Comment on the radiograph

This is an AP radiograph of the left shoulder showing an antero-inferior dislocation of the shoulder. One should look for associated injuries including greater tuberosity fractures, bony Bankart lesions, and glenoid fractures.

Complications of anterior dislocation include: axillary nerve palsy (5–30%), rotator cuff tear (14–63%, increased in the elderly), and greater tuberosity (GT)/glenoid rim fracture (> 20% = fixation).

Structures that may block reduction include: buttonholing through the capsule, biceps tendon, or bony fragments.

Why does the shoulder dislocate? What stops it normally?

The shoulder is a highly mobile joint, but at the expense of stability. When the restraints are overcome, the shoulder will dislocate. There are static and dynamic restraints:
Static restraints:

- Osseous anatomy limited to a third of the head on the glenoid—depth increased by labrum (~50%)
- Negative pressure inside joint
- Capsular thickenings—superior glenohumeral ligament (SGHL)/middle glenohumeral ligament (MGHL)/inferior glenohumeral ligament (IGHL) (most important—hammock analogy)

Dynamic restraints:

- Rotator cuff muscles
- Long head of biceps tendon (LHB)

The A&E staff have tried to reduce this without success—talk me through how you would reduce this dislocation

The patient has his arm externally rotated and abducted with loss of the deltoid contour. If the patient were still sedated I would attempt one further reduction in A&E. If unable to reduce I would mobilize my theatre team and anaesthetist to perform a reduction under general anaesthetic—Flouroscopic (II) control.

- Hippocratic method—foot in axilla on humeral head, traction on abducted arm
- Kocher method of reduction—flex elbow 90°, arm in neutral, then external rotation (ER) slowly until you hear a clunk of reduction. If it does not reduce, flex the shoulder, slowly internal rotate, and fully adduct across the chest (no traction)
- Modified Stimpson = hanging weight prone

If the patient were young I would splint them in an ER position for the first 2 weeks then begin a mobilization programme guided by the physiotherapists.

What is the risk of this shoulder causing problems again?

The re-dislocation rate is proportional to the age at first dislocation.

There is a tendency to be more aggressive in the management of young, first-time dislocations with MRI arthrograms [look for Bankart (+/− bony)/capsular tear/Hill–Sachs lesion] or early examination under anaesthetic (EUA) and arthroscopy to look for and repair Bankart lesions (labral detachment between 3 and 9 o'clock).

What approach would you take for an open reduction?

Deltopectoral. (See answer to previous viva.)

Viva 65

A 30-year-old man falls off his mountain bike and presents to the emergency department complaining of shoulder pain.

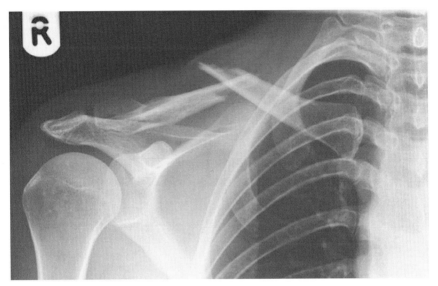

Figure 7.5 A radiograph of a clavicle

Reproduced from Aneel Bhangu, Caroline Lee, and Keith Porter, *Emergencies in Trauma*, 2010, figure 12.5, p. 217, with permission from Oxford University Press.

Describe the radiograph.

Do you know any classifications for such an injury?

How would you manage this patient?

Do you know any recent papers on the management of clavicular fractures?

Describe the radiograph

The radiograph shows a displaced fracture of the middle third of the left clavicle. There is angulation of the fracture and shortening.

Do you know any classifications for such an injury?

Clavicle fractures were classified into thirds by Allman [medial (<5%), middle (80%), lateral (15%)].

Neer revised the Allman classification scheme, with lateral clavicle fractures further divided into three types based on the location of the clavicle fracture in relation to the coracoclavicular ligaments:

- Type I fractures occur lateral to the coracoclavicular ligaments
- Type II fractures occur at the level of coracoclavicular ligaments, with the trapezoid remaining intact with the distal segment
- Type III injuries enter the acromioclavicular (AC) joint

The Neer type II fracture was further divided into type IIA, in which both the conoid and trapezoid ligaments remain attached to the distal fragment, and type IIB, in which the conoid ligament is torn.

How would you manage this patient?

I would initially manage this patient according to ATLS guidelines. He may have sustained a high-energy injury. I would ensure this was an isolated injury to the clavicle. Associated injuries include: subclavian artery injury, brachial plexus injury, and lung injury. I would examine the neurovascular status of the upper limb and the lung fields. I would assess the skin over the fracture. Most middle-third fractures can be managed non-operatively, but this displaced shortened pattern have a higher incidence of non-union (10%), so I would openly reduce and internally fix this fracture with a pre-contoured plate.

Do you know any recent papers on the management of clavicular fractures?

Canadian Orthopaedic Trauma Society (2007). Non-operative treatment compared with plate fixation of displaced midshaft clavicular fractures: a multicentre, randomised clinical trial. *J Bone Joint Surg (Am)* 89, 1–10.

This was a randomized controlled trial with 132 patients; non-operative vs operative midshaft clavicle fracture. The operative group had fewer non-unions (2 vs 7), fewer symptomatic malunions (0 vs 9), quicker time to union (16 vs 28 weeks), and more satisfaction at 1 year. However, the study was not stratified to injury characteristics or subgroups.

Viva 66

Here are some radiographs of a child who has fallen off a swing.

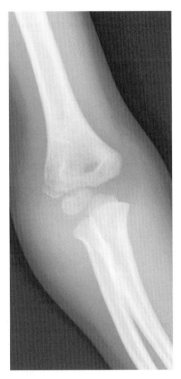

Figure 7.6 An AP and lateral view of an elbow

Describe the injury to me. Can you classify it?

How old do you think the child is? How have you worked that out?

This is an isolated closed injury. How would you manage this definitively?

What are some of the complications of this particular injury?

Describe the injury to me. Can you classify it?

This is an AP radiograph showing a displaced lateral condyle fracture.

Traditionally this injury is classified using the Milch system. This depends on where the fracture exits into the joint relative to the trochlea. It has not been shown to be that useful in terms of guiding management. More important is whether the fracture extends into the joint.

How old do you think the child is? How have you worked that out?

I would estimate the child to be between 3 and 5 years of age. I have based this on the fact that the ossification centres around the child's elbow appear in a standard order:

- Capitellum, 1 year
- Radial head, 3 years
- Medial epicondyle, 5 years
- Trochlea, 7 years
- Olecranon, 9 years
- Lateral epicondyle, 11 years

This is an isolated closed injury. How would you manage this definitively?

My definitive management of this injury would consist of open reduction of the displaced fragment and internal fixation to achieve absolute stability. I would hold my reduction with a partially threaded, small fragment 3.5-mm screw. I would approach the fracture from the lateral side and check my reduction anteriorly avoiding the neurovascular posterior structures. Post-operatively I would protect the soft tissues in a backslab for 3 weeks, and then once they had healed I would start early range of motion exercises.

What are some of the complications of this particular injury?

These fractures have an unusually high rate of non-union for a children's fracture so interfragmentary compression with a lag screw is the optimum treatment. Other complications include angular deformity (cubitus valgus) secondary to a lateral growth arrest. Management of such a deformity remains controversial. In my institution we would only consider an osteotomy at a later date if the deformity gave the child a functional problem. Tardy ulnar nerve palsy is also a late, and luckily rare, complication.

Viva 67

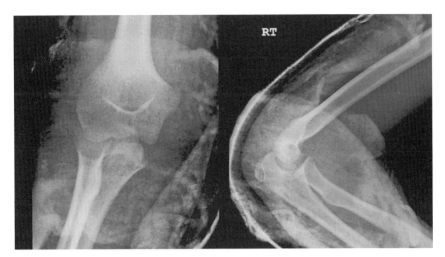

Figure 7.7 An AP and lateral view of an elbow

Describe the radiographs and explain your initial management.

What other injuries can be associated with this diagnosis?

How would you do a closed reduction for a dislocated elbow?

When would an open reduction be required?

For the above X-rays what approach would be used if open reduction were required?

When would you see this patient in clinic and when would you start mobilizing the elbow?

Describe the radiographs and explain your initial management

AP and oblique radiographs of an elbow in a skeletally immature patient. There is a bone fragment in the joint space, which probably represents a medial epicondyle fracture. It is highly likely this elbow dislocated and, as it relocated, the medial epicondyle has flipped into the joint.

Initial management would be according to ATLS protocol, ruling out other injuries and making sure the patient is stable. Initial elbow management entails examination including a neurovascular assessment.

What other injuries can be associated with this diagnosis?

- Bone injuries
  - Medial epicondyle (most common associated fracture)
  - Lateral epicondyle
  - Radius head
  - Avulsion of the olecranon
  - Coronoid fracture

Neurovascular injuries

  - Ulnar nerve at risk with associated medial epicondyle avulsions (most common neuropathy)
  - Median nerve entrapment has been reported in the literature
  - Brachial artery injury can occur

How would you do a closed reduction for a dislocated elbow?

The most common elbow dislocation is posterior or posterolateral and I would reduce this by:

- Inline traction to correct coronal displacement
- Supination to clear the coronoid beneath the trochlea
- Flexion of the elbow while placing pressure on the tip of the olecranon

Post-reduction radiographs would be required for re-evaluation and, if needed, a post-reduction computerized tomography (CT) scan to confirm the associated fracture.

When would an open reduction be required?

- Open dislocation of the elbow
- Failure to achieve a concentric joint reduction
- Incarcerated bone fragment in the joint, e.g. medial epicondyle
- Unstable elbow post reduction
- Nerve deficit, e.g. ulnar nerve in the presence of a medial epicondyle fracture

For the above X-rays what approach would be used if open reduction were required?

Elbow medial approach.

When would you see this patient in clinic and when would you start mobilizing the elbow?

If a concentric joint reduction is achieved and the elbow is stable, I would review the patient in a week's time with an X-ray on arrival. I would start physiotherapy and elbow mobilization in 2 weeks from the injury to avoid stiffness.

Viva 68

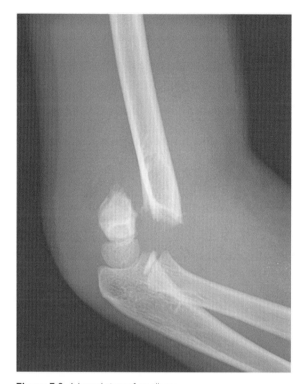

Figure 7.8 A lateral view of an elbow

Describe the X-rays. How would you initially manage this patient?

What neurovascular injuries could be associated with this fracture?

It is midnight and the patient has got a pink, pulseless hand. How would you manage the patient?

If the hand were blue and pulseless, would your management differ? What would you do?

What are the concepts of closed reduction?

What are the most common causes of an inability to achieve a satisfactory closed reduction?

Post-operatively the patient develops weakness in the median nerve distribution. How would you manage this? If this were the ulnar distribution, would your management differ?

Is cubitus varus or cubitus valgus better and why? How would you manage both?

Describe the X-rays and how would you initially manage this patient?

This is an elbow X-ray of a skeletally immature patient showing an off-ended supracondylar (SC) fracture. This is an extension type and can be classified as type III according to the Gratland classification.

The standard of care is surgical management with closed reduction and percutaneous pin fixation.

What neurovascular injuries could be associated with this fracture?

Brachial artery. In most situations it is stretched over the displaced fracture fragments. Direct injury may occur where the artery can be contused or may have sustained an intimal injury with development of an aneurysm or delayed occlusive thrombus. Additionally, the brachial artery may be partially lacerated or completely transected.

Neurovascular injury can be predicted based on the direction of displacement

- Extension type
  - Posterolateral displacement: associated with median and anterior interosseous nerve injuries
  - Posteromedial displacement: associated with radial nerve injuries
- Flexion type
  - Commonly associated with ulnar nerve injuries

It is midnight and the patient has got a pink, pulseless hand. How would you manage the patient?

According to the British Society for Children's Orthopaedic Surgery (BSCOS), a perfused limb does not require brachial artery exploration whether or not the radial pulse is present.

To date, the American Academy of Orthopaedic Surgeons (AAOS) has been unable to establish definitive clinical guidance owing to the paucity of high-level scientific evidence. Following reduction and stabilization the vascular status is reevaluated. If the pulses are restored, there will be no need for vascular intervention. If the pulse does not return but the hand remains well perfused, optimal management is less clear. Some surgeons advocate immediate vascular exploration while others propose inpatient observation for 24–48 h with frequent neurovascular monitoring. If perfusion becomes compromised during observation, vascular exploration is necessary. There is evidence in the literature to support that watchful waiting can result in good functional outcome and normal extremity development with very small incidence of surgical exploration being required.

If the hand were blue and pulseless, would your management differ? What would you do?

In the setting of a poorly perfused, pulseless limb emergency operative reduction and fixation should be performed. If perfusion to the extremity does not improve after reduction, immediate open vascular exploration and possible reconstruction is indicated.

What are the concepts of closed reduction?

Extension type is the most common and the concepts are as follows:

1. Displacement is corrected in the coronal and horizontal planes before the sagittal plane
2. Hyperextension of the elbow with longitudinal traction attempting to obtain apposition
3. Valgus or varus force may be needed to address a varus or valgus deformity, respectively
4. Flexion of the elbow is done while applying a posterior force to the distal fragment

What are the most common causes of an inability to achieve a satisfactory closed reduction?

- Interposition of the brachialis muscle, with buttonholing of the metaphyseal spike through the muscle
- Entrapment of the brachial artery
- Entrapment of neurological structures, such as the median nerve
- Interposition of the periosteum or joint capsule within the fracture site

Post-operatively the patient develops weakness in the median nerve distribution. How would you manage this? If this were the ulnar distribution, would your management differ?

Median nerve deficit post closed reduction may indicate entrapment of the median nerve at the fracture site. Ulnar nerve injury post closed reduction and pinning can be iatrogenic following the use of a medial wire with a crossed wire configuration. According to the BSCOS guidelines 'If there is concern over iatrogenic injury then a thorough assessment with consultant input is required for consideration of nerve exploration'.

Is cubitus varus or cubitus valgus better and why? How would you manage both?

Cubitus varus (gunstock deformity) is caused by fracture malunion and is usually a cosmetic issue with few functional limitations. It could be avoided by aiming to achieve a Baumann angle similar to the contralateral arm intra-operatively. This can be managed with supracondylar osteotomy of the humerus. Cubitus valgus is caused by fracture malunion and can lead to tardy ulnar nerve palsy. There is evidence in the literature that the extent of valgus deformity may not progress after fracture healing. Ulnar neuropathy owing to traumatic cubitus valgus deformity can be treated with anterior subcutaneous ulnar transposition.

Viva 69

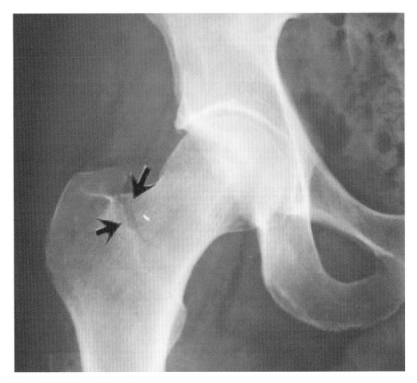

Figure 7.9 A lateral view of a knee

Describe the radiograph.

What other injuries could be associated with this injury?

Describe the bundles that form the injured structure. What is the blood supply?

Briefly, what clinical tests would you do in clinic to examine for the injured structure?

Why is gait assessment essential in patients with a chronic injury?

If this is an isolated injury, how would you treat it?

Describe the radiograph

A lateral knee radiograph showing a posterior avulsion of a bone fragment, possibly reflecting bone avulsion of the posterior cruciate ligament (PCL).

What other injuries could be associated with this injury?

Posterolateral corner (PLC) injuries, multi-ligamentous knee injuries, and knee dislocation. Treatment may be compromised if other injuries are not recognized.

Describe the bundles that form the injured structure. What is the blood supply?

The PCL has two major bundles, functionally described as the anterolateral and posteromedial bands. The first is the larger and accounts for 85% of the cross-sectional area of the ligament. It is this band that is reconstructed in single-bundle reconstructions. It is tight in flexion and lax in extension, while the posteromedial bundle is tight in extension and lax in flexion.
Blood supply is through branches of the middle geniculate artery and fat pad.

Briefly, what clinical tests would you do in clinic to examine for the injured structure?

A careful examination of the neurological and vascular status is mandatory. The common peroneal nerve is at risk from injury to the lateral complex. Posterior knee dislocation is associated with the highest rate of popliteal artery tear.

- Posterior sag sign: with the patient lying supine with hips and knees flexed to 90°
- Posterior drawer test: at 90° of knee flexion. Extent of posterior subluxation can be graded I–III according to the relation of the medial tibial plateau to the anterior aspect of the medial femoral condyle. Posterior sag of grade 2 or 3 almost invariably indicates a degree of damage to the posterolateral structures
- Quadriceps active test: positive if anterior reduction of the tibia onto the femur occurs with attempted extension of the knee from 90° flexion
- Dial test (supine or prone position): increased ER at 30° but not at 90° of knee flexion is indicative of isolated rupture of the PLC. A positive test at both 30° and 90° suggests rupture of both
- Varus/valgus stress: laxity at 0° indicates Medial collateral ligament (MCL)/lateral collateral ligament (LCL) and PCL injury. Laxity at 30° alone indicates MCL/LCL injury

Why is gait assessment essential in patients with a chronic injury?

Examination of gait is essential as it may demonstrate an obvious varus thrust of the knee. Any suggestion of physiological varus of the knee should result in careful assessment including full radiographs of the leg and a decision made on whether a valgus tibial osteotomy is necessary to decrease the tension in the soft-tissue structures of the lateral side of the knee. Altering the tibial slope is an important concept in the management of chronic PCL-deficient knee. An opening wedge osteotomy to increase the tibial slope will prevent posterior translation of the tibia.

If this is an isolated injury, how would you treat it?

Bony avulsion of the insertion of the PCL into the back of the tibia is an indication for early operative treatment using the posterior or the posteromedial approach to the knee.

Viva 70

This is the C-ray of a young athlete complaining of right hip pain after a marathon.

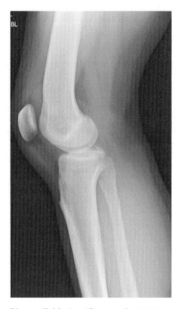

Figure 7.10 An AP view of right hip

What fracture types would you expect and what type is shown in the above X-ray?

Several characteristics identified on imaging have been shown to influence the bio-mechanical stability of the fracture. Can you elaborate?

What is the blood supply to the femoral head?

What variables can contribute to femoral head osteonecrosis?

How would you treat this injury?

If this fracture were displaced, would you do a closed or an open reduction?

On attempting closed reduction can you describe an attempted manoeuvre for closed reduction?

What approach can you use for open reduction?

For how long would you follow a patient with a displaced fracture and what is the reported incidence of osteonecrosis?

What fracture types would you expect and what type is shown in the above X-ray?

Fracture of the femoral neck secondary to repetitive loading of bone can be of two types:

- Compression side (inferior-medial neck)
- Tension side (superior-lateral neck)

The above X-ray is an AP view of a skeletally mature patient showing a fracture on the tension side.

Several characteristics identified on imaging have been shown to influence the biomechanical stability of the fracture. Can you elaborate?

The verticality of the fracture line in the coronal plane should be assessed. Pauwels first recognized the significance of high-angle fractures in the 1930s. He established a descriptive classification scheme that helps determine fracture stability based on the 'Pauwels angle'. A femoral neck fracture line < 30° from the horizontal plane is Pauwels Type I; a fracture with an angle between 30 and 50° is Pauwels Type II; and an angle of > 50° is categorized as a Pauwels Type III fracture. Increased verticality of the fracture decreases the load shared through the fracture fragments resulting in a biomechanically unstable pattern.

What is the blood supply to the femoral head?

The blood supply comes from three main sources: the medial femoral circumflex artery, the lateral femoral circumflex artery, and the obturator artery.

- The medial femoral circumflex artery is the largest contributor to the blood supply of the femoral head, especially its superolateral aspect. The lateral epiphyseal artery complex originates from it and courses along the posterosuperior aspect of the femoral neck before supplying the femoral head
- The lateral femoral circumflex artery gives rise to the inferior metaphyseal artery by way of the ascending branch and supplies the majority of the inferoanterior aspect of the femoral head
- The obturator artery provides small and variable amounts of the blood supply to the femoral head through the ligamentum teres

What variables can contribute to femoral head osteonecrosis?

- Vascular damage from the initial femoral neck fracture
- The quality of the reduction or fixation of the fracture

How would you treat this injury?

Operative management is recommended for non-displaced impacted fractures. Anatomical reduction and stable internal fixation are paramount for a good outcome. Non-operative management of a non-displaced femoral neck fracture is associated with higher complication rates and an increased risk of displacement, especially when the fracture is on the tension side.

If this fracture were displaced, would you do a closed or an open reduction?

There is no gold standard. Proceed with closed or open reduction for displaced femoral neck fractures in young adults as long as anatomic reduction is achieved.

On attempting closed reduction can you describe an attempted manoeuvre for closed reduction?

Leadbetter first described in 1939 the manoeuvre to reduce femoral neck fractures. The affected leg is flexed to 45° with slight abduction and then extended with internal rotation while longitudinal traction is applied. Anatomic reduction is verified with fluoroscopy in the AP and lateral view.

What approach can you use for open reduction?

Traditionally two different surgical approaches have been utilized for internal fixation: the Watson Jones (antero-lateral) and the modified Smith-Peterson (anterior) approaches.

For how long would you follow a patient with a displaced fracture and what is the reported incidence of osteonecrosis?

The incidence has been documented to be as high as 86%. Osteonecrosis of the femoral head can present anywhere between 6 months and many years after the initial injury; however, most cases will present within 2 years. For this reason, I would follow the patient up for at least 2 years post-operatively looking for signs of osteonecrosis, both clinically and radiologically.

Part 4   **Adult Pathology**

Chapter 8   **Foot and Ankle**

Viva 71

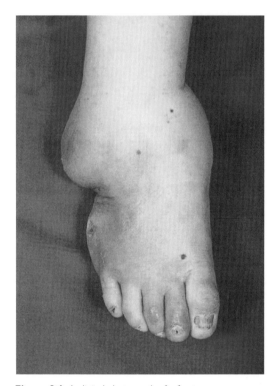

Figure 8.1 A clinical photograph of a foot.

Reproduced from Murray Longmore, Ian Wilkinson, Edward Davidson, Alexander Foulkes, and Ahmad Mafi, *Oxford Handbook of Clinical Medicine*, figure 2, p. 205, 2010, with permission from Oxford University Press.

What do you see?

How does it evolve?

What are the principles of treating this condition?

What do you see?

This is a clinical photograph of a grossly deformed foot and ankle.

Charcot arthropathy is a severe destructive arthropathy that can occur in any patient with a sensory disturbance. Over 90% of cases in the UK are related to diabetic neuropathy (it occurs in 1% of diabetics who have had the disease for 12 years). The other causes can be thought of along the course of the sensory neurological system from peripheral to central:

- Alcoholic peripheral neuropathy
- Post-traumatic sensory deficits
- Tertiary syphilis
- Spina bifida
- Hereditary motor and sensory neuropathy
- Congenital insensation to pain

How does it evolve?

The pathophysiology is not fully understood, but is generally thought to be caused by a combination of neurotraumatic and neurovascular factors. It is probably initiated by trauma; however, often no injury can be recollected by the patient. There is rapid destruction of the joint surface and demineralization, which appears to be caused by osteoclast overactivity, bone vascular shunting, and bone breakdown. This leads to loss of normal foot architecture. This phase is often said to be painless, but there is usually some pain (often less than may be expected). Healing begins and there is usually bony union with joint incongruity and foot deformity.

Eichenholz has staged this process:

- Collapse. The foot becomes painful, swollen (oedematous), and warm (erythematous). X-rays may show a fracture/fractures or dislocation. This stage can be difficult to differentiate from an acute infection. Over the following weeks the oedema and erythema settle, although the foot can continue to change shape (unless protected) as the bone continues to fragment. As a general rule, if the skin is intact think Charcot; if the skin is broken it is most likely infection; the history will often lead you
- Coalescence. The foot continues to settle and starts to stiffen up and the deformities become fixed. X-rays show coalescence of small fracture fragments and adsorption of fine bone debris
- Consolidation. Over many months the oedema and erythema completely settle. The X-rays show consolidation and remodelling of fracture fragments (as a rough guide forefoot 6 months, midfoot 12 months, hindfoot 18 months)

What are the principles of treating this condition?

1. Prevention: optimum management of co-morbidities (diabetes)
2. Early diagnosis: high index of suspicion, loss of protective sensation (use Semmes–Weinstein monofilaments 5.02)
3. In the early phase support the foot to maintain foot shape and prevent gross deformity. Weight bearing should be restricted. This must be done with care because often patients lack protective sensation and casts and braces can cause ulceration (total contact casting)
4. Once consolidation is well underway the foot can be returned to some form of shoe wear [this can take many months (12–18)]. Often lifelong, specially made orthotics will be required. Patients must be made aware of the risks of skin breakdown and inspect their feet closely each day

Viva 72

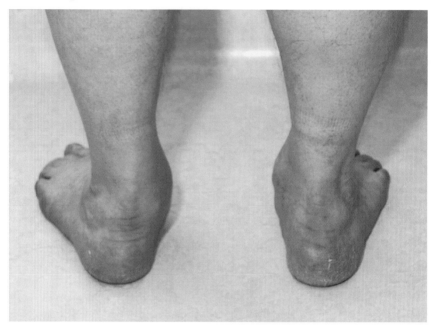

Figure 8.2 A clinical photograph of a patient's ankles and feet.

Reproduced from Raashid Luqmani, Theodore Pincus, and Maarten Boers, *Rheumatoid Arthritis* (Oxford Rheumatology Library), 2010, Figure 11.6, p. 138, with permission from Oxford University Press.

Describe this picture.

What are the stages of this condition and how are they managed?

Describe this picture

This is a picture of a plano-valgus foot. There is the 'too many toes' sign. Pes planus can be congenital or acquired. The most common cause of adult acquired flat foot is tibialis posterior tendon dysfunction. The tibialis posterior tendon is the main invertor of the hindfoot. It also acts as an elevator of the midfoot (sling) as it inserts into the navicular, plantar cuneiforms, and second, third, and fourth metatarsal (MT) bases.

The condition is most often seen in middle-aged women whose body morphology aided by gravity tests the tendon as it is starting to age.

What are the stages of this condition and how are they managed?

The tendon can become inflamed, painful, and swollen. The foot does not initially change shape and patients are still able to single-leg tiptoe, although they quickly fatigue (Johnson Stage 1). Some patients settle with enforced rest in a supportive brace or cast.

As the tendon degenerates it lengthens. The foot changes shape with the hindfoot going into valgus. Patients are no longer able to single-leg tiptoe (often the pain over the tib post may have settled, especially if the tendon has completely ruptured). If the hindfoot is still flexible (Johnson Stage 2), this can be treated with either orthotics to help support the foot and medial arch, or surgery. Surgery involves reinforcing the tibialis posterior tendon (TPT) with a flexor digitorum longus (FDL) tendon transfer. This reconstruction is then protected by bringing the hindfoot into neutral alignment with a medial sliding calcaneal osteotomy. The tibialis anterior (TA) occasionally needs to be released (percutaneously) as if the hindfoot has been in valgus for some time it will have tightened preventing full correction to neutral.

If the valgus hindfoot deformity is fixed (Johnson Stage 3), reconstruction is not achievable. The subtalar joint is degenerate. Surgical treatments involve a talonavicular and subtalar fusion or a formal triple arthrodesis.

Myerson added a fourth stage when the deformity led to significant ankle arthritis secondary to valgus strain.

Viva 73

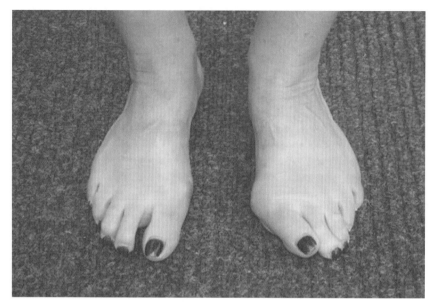

Figure 8.3 A clinical photograph of a patient's feet.

What is this?

What do you look at on the X-ray?

What are the treatment options?

What is this?

This is a clinical picture of a foot with hallux valgus and a large inflamed bunion.

- This condition is common
- Most often found in middle-aged women (also teenage girls with a strong family history)
- Occurs in females four times as often as in males
- Not common in communities where no formal shoewear is worn

Aetiology

There is a strong genetic component (Family History +ve); inappropriate shoewear plays a role.

Pathology

1. Capsule stretches medially
2. Structures tighten laterally (adductor hallucis)
3. Sesamoids stay with second MT attached via intermalleolar ligament (IML)
4. MT head slips medially off sesamoids via erosion of the crista and hallux deviates laterally
5. Abnormal muscle pull of extensor hallucis longus and brevis increases the deformity
6. As the first ray effectively shortens and defunctions, patients start getting transfer metatarsalgia. The second metatarsophalangeal (MTP) joint can become inflamed and synovitic leading to clawing of the second toe and subluxation of the joint

Clinical symptoms

Pain caused by the inflamed bunion; crossover of toes causing difficulty with shoewear; transfer metatarsalgia as first ray defunctions; patients often complain of the appearance.

What do you look at on the X-ray?

Look at:

- The severity of hallux valgus [(HV) angle and intermetatarsal angle (IMA)]
- The state of joint and articular congruity, position of sesamoids
- Second ray/subluxation of second MTP joint
- HV interphalangeus (HVIP): IMA < 9°; HVA < 15°; interphalangeal angle (IPA) < 10°; distal metatarsal articular angle (DMAA) < 10° (discredited on most papers as not reproducible)
- Sesamoid shift: grade 0–3 (0, none; 1, < 50%; 2, > 50%; 3, > 100%)
- Metatarsus prima varus = angle between long axis medial cuneiform and first MT
- Natural cascade: first and second MTs same length; third 3 mm shorter; fourth 6 mm shorter; fifth 12 mm shorter

What are the treatment options?

- Non-operative: information sheet; shoewear modification (wide toe box); bunion pads and toe spacers; avoidance of high heels; analgesics
- Operative: indications = failure of non-operative management or worsening pain (not for cosmetic reasons)

Surgical options are individual choices. In general, if the IMA is < 12° then a distal osteotomy may be acceptable (chevron preferred). If the IMA is > 13° then a proximal or Scarf osteotomy would be better. If the HV is marked (IMA > 20°) or there is HVIP then an Akin osteotomy can be performed to give a more powerful correction. If there is osteoarthritis (OA) in the first MTP joint a fusion should be recommended.

Viva 74

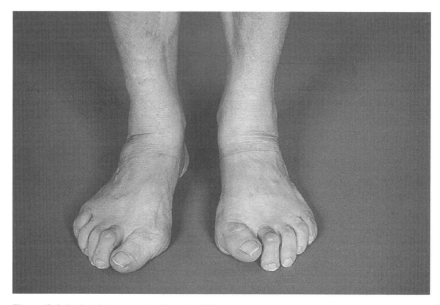

Figure 8.4 A clinical photograph of a patient's feet.

Reproduced from C. Bulstrode et al., *Oxford Textbook of Trauma and Orthopaedics* second edition, 2011, figure 10.2.3, p. 795, with permission from Oxford University Press.

What are the common deformities seen in the foot with rheumatoid arthritis (RA)?

How do these deformities occur?

Describe how you would manage this patient.

What are the common deformities seen in the foot with rheumatoid arthritis (RA)?

RA commonly causes foot deformities. It can affect the forefoot, midfoot, and hindfoot. RA causes synovitis. The inflammatory response within the joint and the subsequent release of pro-teases and collagenases destroy hyaline cartilage and cause periarticular attenuation of soft-tissue capsuloligamentous structures. This leads to instability and abnormal mechanics; secondary OA often leads to further deformity. The incidence of rheumatoid foot deformities has dropped dramatically with modern disease-modifying anti-rheumatoid drugs (DMARDs).

How do these deformities occur?

Forefoot deformity

1. Synovitis in the MTP joints leads to attenuation of soft tissues, in particular the plantar plate. Pain from the synovitis and disruption of the plantar plate allows the toes to claw up with hyperextended MTP joints and flexed interphalangeal joints
2. As the MTP joints sublux with disruption of the plantar plates (attached to the plantar fascia and fat pads, which normally cushion MT heads from direct pressure) the cushioning fat pads are pulled forwards
3. The MT heads become prominent in the sole of the foot—predisposing to callosities, skin ulceration, and breakdown (feeling of 'walking on pebbles')
4. HV is often present but doesn't usually cause a problem

Midfoot deformity

Involvement of the midtarsal joint leads to collapse of the long arch. This can be secondary to failure of the TPT, which normally acts as a sling for the midfoot.

Hindfoot deformity

Tibialis posterior insufficiency and gradual disruption of the talocalcaneal interosseous (IO) ligament (important stabilizer of the subtalar joint) lead to progressive valgus deformity of the hindfoot and collapse of the medial arch.

Describe how you would manage this patient

This would include a multidisciplinary approach. These patients have multiple other problems involving their musculoskeletal system as well as other co-morbidities. Often despite considerable deformity, the feet may not be very disabling. In general it is sensible to address the more proximal joint problems first (hip/knee). It is important to work up rheumatoid patients prior to interventions as they have a higher risk of all complications—infection (~5%)/wound-healing problems.

1. Medical optimization—multidisciplinary team with rheumatologists regarding normal medication
   - Methotrexate to continue
   - Anti-tumour necrosis factor (TNF)—(plan surgery in between doses)
   - Decrease steroids as much as possible; dose peri-operatively
2. Anaesthetic input—cervical spine (flexion/extension views)/positioning and padding
3. Other joints—upper limb function (difficulty with crutches/sticks); physiotherapy and occupational therapy input

Management of foot disease

Non-operative management consists of: custom-made orthotics to accommodate the deformity/padded heels/locked or limited motion ankle foot orthosis (with valgus corrective T strap)/information sheets/medical optimization.

Operative: the goal is a stable pain-free plantargrade foot. The trend now is towards joint preservation. Historically first MTP joint fusion with excision of lesser MT heads. Now consider Scarf, Weils, or Stainsbys.

1. HV—arthrodesis MTP joint (10° dorsiflex/10° valgus)
2. Lesser toes—if destroyed joints—resection of MT heads (Fowler's) or proximal interphalangeal joint correction and fusion. If joints are okay or in a younger patient, Weil's shortening osteotomy of MT heads, which allows reduction of MTP joints and return of fat pad into the sole of the foot
3. Midfoot—talonavicular fusion +/− calcaneocuboid fusion
4. Hindfoot—triple fusion
5. Ankle—fusion vs arthroplasty (RA is one of the best indications for ankle arthroplasty as these patients are low demand and have other joints affected)
   • Not enough data to indicate whether fusion or replacement is to be preferred for patients in whom either procedure would be an option
   • At ~10 years clinical success rates appear similar [systematic review—paper by Haddad (2007) *Journal of Bone and Joint Surgery* (American volume) found 70% satisfactory results after both procedures]
   • Non-union rate for ankle fusion was 10%—arthroplasty survival rate 77% at 10 years

Viva 75

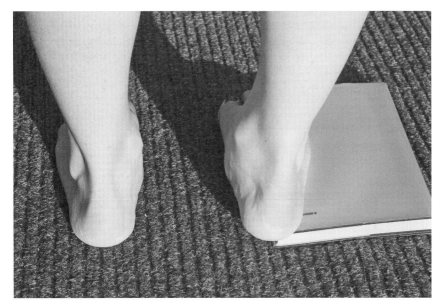

Figure 8.5 A clinical test.

Describe what you see and how you would assess the patient?

What are the causes of this deformity?

How does a patient present and what are the principles of treatment?

Describe what you see and how you would assess the patient?

The patient is standing with the lateral border of the right foot on a book. This is the Coleman block test and shows that a varus deformity of the hindfoot is correctable. This indicates that the subtalar joint is mobile and the varus hindfoot deformity is driven by excess plantarflexion of the first ray. I would expect there also to be clawing of the toes with hyperextension of the metatarsophalangeal joints and flexion of the interphalangeal joints. If this is unilateral it is caused by a spinal cord tumour until proven otherwise. I would like to see the patient walk to check if they have a broad-based ataxic gait. I would like to have a look at their back and perform a lower-leg neurological examination. I would inspect their hands for any intrinsic wasting. I would ask the patient what troubles they get from their feet so we can decide on an appropriate management plan.

What are the causes of this deformity?

These can be congenital or acquired [hereditary motor sensory neuropathy (HMSN) is by far the most common].

* Congenital: idiopathic/arthrogrypotic/residual clubfoot
* Acquired:
  * Neurological
  * Brain—Friedreich's ataxia
* Spinal cord (SC)—pina bifida, polio, syrinx
* peripheral nervous system (PNS)—HMSN [Charcot–Marie–Tooth CMT)]
  * Muscular—muscular dystrophies
  * Traumatic
  * Neoplastic

CMT/HMSN

Lots of subtypes described as genetic knowledge improves, but there are two main types:

Early: Type 1, demyelinating type; autosomal dominant in 50% with six subtypes; ages 5–15 years old; loss of reflexes; abnormal nerve conduction studies (NCS); hands involved

Later: Type 2, axonal autosomal dominant with 12 subtypes; ages 15–20 years old; NCS are normal

How does a patient present and what are the principles of management?

Patients present with deformity and instability, with repeated ankle sprains and painful callosities (secondary to clawing). History is important (is there a family history?).

Patients need a full assessment including: a neurological assessment, whole-body X-rays, magnetic resonance imaging (MRI) (spine), and NCS+/– electromyography.

They should be referred to a neurologist for investigation of the cause and often a genetic consultation is helpful.

Orthopaedic treatment is best categorised by the ability to correct the deformity.

* Non-operative:
  * Stretching; physio; serial casts, in kids +/– orthotics (corrective—if flexible, e.g. lateral heel wedge) vs accommodative (if fixed)
* Operative (soft-tissue or bony or both):
  * Aims of treatment are to achieve plantargrade, stable foot that moves and is pain-free
  * Decision is based on the age of patient and whether deformity is flexible or fixed

Chapter 9   Knee

Viva 76

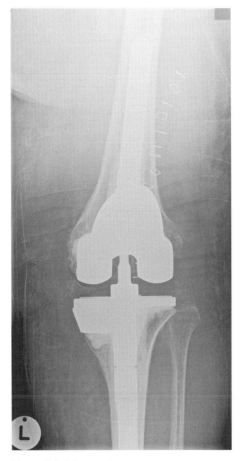

Figure 9.1 A knee replacement.

What implants do you use for revision total knee replacements (TKRs)?

You are passed a hinged prosthesis. What are the benefits and disadvantages of this type of component?

If you were to revise a unicompartmental knee replacement (UKR) what implant would you choose?

If you had a patient with a PS knee with a complete medial collateral ligament (MCL) disruption and dislocation, what implant choice might you make?

What implants do you use for revision total knee replacements (TKRs)?

This question is aimed at exploring your understanding of pre-op planning based on the individual requirements of the clinical case. The range of implants or system I use would depend on the clinical situation.

Possibilities include: primary TKR, posterior-stabilized (PS), super-stabilized, rotating hinge, with stems +/− augments, and tumour prosthesis. Whenever faced with a revision situation it is also prudent to consider both amputation and arthrodesis as options.

You are passed a hinged prosthesis. What are the benefits and disadvantages of this type of component?

These implants are used in ligament insufficiency and/or cases with major bone loss. The problem with increasingly constrained implants is transmission of high forces across the bone–cement–implant interface, which can lead to premature loosening.

If you were to revise a unicompartmental knee replacement (UKR) what implant would you choose?

Ideally I would use a primary TKR implant. If there has been some tibial loosening and bone loss, a stemmed implant, possibly with augments, may be required.

If you had a patient with a PS knee with a complete medial collateral ligament (MCL) disruption and dislocation what implant choice might you make?

Most likely I would require a rotating hinge stemmed system.

Viva 77

You see a woman 6 months following a TKR. She is complaining of pain.

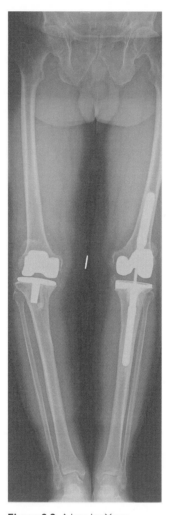

Figure 9.2 A long leg X-ray.

What are the most common causes of pain following a TKR?

How would you investigate and manage this patient?

The blood tests show raised CRP and ESR, and the aspirate grows coagulase-negative, Gram-positive cocci after 5 days. How do you manage this?

What are the most common causes of pain following a TKR?

This is still fairly early after a TKR and many patients still have pain that continues to resolve at this stage.

- Infection—this may not be most common cause but it is the most important to exclude
- Patello-femoral problems
- Component malposition (overhang, malalignment, poor cementing)
- Loosening
- Complex regional pain syndrome (CRPS)
- Instability
- Dual pathology (hip arthritis)

How would you investigate and manage this patient?

I would take a careful history. This needs to include an assessment of the patient prior to the TKR, the intra-operative and immediate post-operative care, including wound healing, length of stay, and any reported complications. Has there been a period when the knee was any good? How is the knee now (start-up pain?). Are there any co-morbidities—infection is more likely with diabetes mellitus (DM), rheumatoid arthritis, steroids, etc.

I would examine the patient, looking for an effusion/haemarthrosis, the alignment, soft tissues, any evidence of CRPS, the range of motion (ROM), patello-femoral (PF) tracking, any patella clunk, balance, flex/extension mismatch, tender areas, and the patient's hips.

Investigations would include: X-ray, looking for component sizing, tibial overhang, femoral sizing, PF joint overstuffing, patella subluxation, loosening/infection, #'s, and heterotopic ossification.

I would perform blood tests for C-reactive protein (CRP) and erythrocyte sedimentation rate (ESR).

I would consider a bone scan, though it is of no help at 6 months.

A computerized tomography (CT) scan may help assess rotation of components.

Finally, I would consider aspiration/biopsy if concerned regarding infection.

Arthroscopy may be of use if a treatable cause is identified.

The blood tests show raised CRP and ESR, and the aspirate grows coagulase-negative, Gram-positive cocci after 5 days. How do you manage this?

This seems to be a prosthetic infection with *Staphylococcus epidermidis*. I would discuss with the patient the diagnosis, the various treatment options, and the possible outcomes (function, further surgery, best- and worst-case scenarios). The treatment options would depend on the patient's physiological status and wishes.

The surgical options at this stage are either debride and retain (DAIR) or revision (single-stage or two-stage). I would also seek advice from a microbiologist.

Viva 78

A 25-year-old football player has sustained a twisting injury to his right knee. He is referred by a colleague with a magnetic resonance imaging (MRI) scan showing an anterior cruciate ligament (ACL) rupture and a bucket handle tear of the medial meniscus.

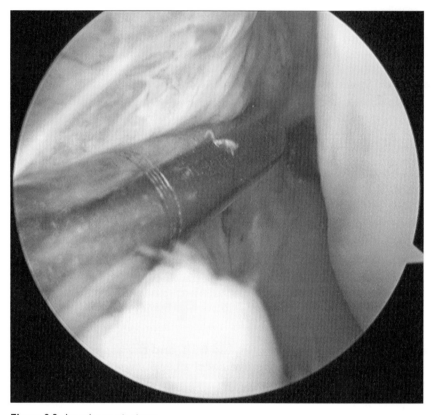

Figure 9.3 An arthroscopic picture.

What is important in your assessment of this patient?

The patient has recurrent instability and has been unable to return to football. Examination confirms ACL injury and he has a full ROM. What are the management options?

You have decided to reconstruct the ACL. What graft would you use?

What is important in your assessment of this patient?

The history of the injury, specifically how long ago. Symptoms since the injury. Continued instability, locking, significant subsequent injuries [is this an acute medial meniscus (MM) tear?]. Occupation and sporting aspirations. Expectations. Past medical history, including co-morbidities, e.g. DM, collagen disorder, previous surgery.

On examination: fixed flexion deformity (FFD), comfortable ROM, signs of meniscal pathology, signs of ACL disruption, e.g. Lachman and pivot shift (both can be negative in cases with bucket handle meniscal tears as the displaced meniscal tissue provides some increased stability to the knee). Evidence of any other ligament injury. If they have had significant secondary injuries it can be useful to get a fresh MRI scan to assess for secondary meniscal injuries.

The patient has recurrent instability and has been unable to return to football. Examination confirms ACL injury and he has a full ROM. What are the management options?

There are two factors to address here: treatment of the ACL and treatment of the meniscal injury. ACL injuries can be managed non-operatively and operatively. An assessment needs to be made of the risks of further meniscal injuries as this predicts the likelihood of early osteoarthritis. High meniscal injury risk factors include: young age, level 1 sports, high number of hours of participation in sport per week, and previous meniscal injury. In view of this patient's history, I would recommend an ACL reconstruction.

The MM injury requires surgery. The key decision is to repair or resect the unstable meniscal tissue. Factors that would make you wish to repair the meniscus would be recent injury (and easily reducible), red–red or red–white zone injury, concurrent ACL injury (increased healing rates), and young age (it is worth noting also that the results of lateral meniscal repairs are better than MM repairs). My choice would be to perform an arthroscopic ACL reconstruction and concurrent meniscal repair if indicated.

You have decided to reconstruct the ACL. What graft would you use?

Have a view yourself. I would use a four-strand hamstring graft with suspensory femoral fixation (endobutton) and round-headed cannulated interference (RCI) screw fixation on the tibial side, but also be aware of the other options, there are advantages and disadvantages.

- Autograft:
  - Hamstring tendons: good long-term results and low donor site morbidity but slower healing into bony tunnels
  - Patella tendon: good long-term results, but donor site morbidity
- Allograft:
  - Typically tibialis anterior: no donor site morbidity but infection risk and, depending on sterilization techniques, less strong; also expensive
- Artificial: avoid

Viva 79

This is a picture of a 67-year-old lady with a painful knee . The pain has been increasing over the past 3 years. She is otherwise fit and well.

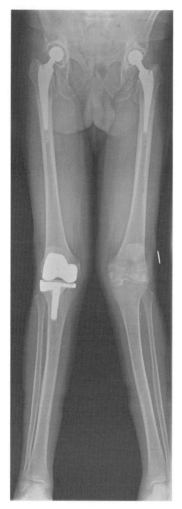

Figure 9.4 A radiograph showing a valgus knee.

How would you manage this patient?

How would you consent the patient for a TKR?

Describe your plan for surgery in this case.

How would you manage this patient?

I would establish from the history more about her pain, disability, and what treatment she has so far received. On examination I would look at the nature of the deformity, if it is correctable, the integrity of the MCL, patella tracking, and neurological status common peroneal nerve (CPN). I would examine her hip and foot. I would arrange some radiographs including standing antero-posterior (AP), lateral, Von Rosenberg, and skyline patella views. The skyline view can be useful with valgus deformities. I may want a long leg film.

Treatment would include maximizing conservative measures; if this failed I would discuss with the patient knee arthroplasty surgery (lateral unicompartmental/total).

How would you consent the patient for a TKR?

I would describe the natural history of the condition. I would describe the procedure as well as alternative treatments. I would describe the anticipated prognosis and success rates of the surgery in terms of pain relief, functional outcome, and longevity. I would explain the risks and complications of the surgery, including general risks and specific risks for TKRs as well as specific risks for TKRs in valgus knee patients.

Describe your plan for surgery in this case

Correct indications met
Patient fully consented
Antibiotic prophylaxis
Choice of implant
Choice of approach

Principles of bony cuts, especially rotation of femoral component. How will I assess this (hypoplastic or wear on posterior lateral femoral condyle make posterior referencing inaccurate)?
What will I do with the patella?
Soft-tissue balancing (sequence of releases).
Implantation of prosthesis and cementing technique.
Drain?
Post-operative management. Deep vein thrombosis prophylaxis.
Follow-up.

Viva 80

A 50-year-old carpenter has had two previous knee arthroscopies for medial-sided knee pain at another hospital. He tells you that his knee was washed out and some of the 'shock-absorbing cartilage' was trimmed. His symptoms have not improved and he has come to you to see if the 'shock-absorbing cartilage' can be repaired.

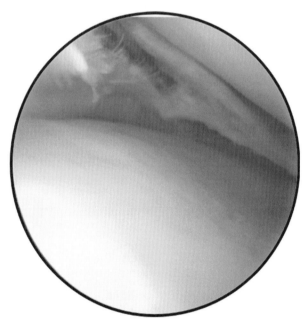

Figure 9.5 An arthroscopic picture.

What pathology does this arthroscopic view of the medial compartment of the knee show?

How can meniscal tears be described?

What is the main function of the meniscus and what clinical relevance does this have with regard to meniscectomy?

What are the other functions of the meniscus?

What clinical relevance does the blood supply of the meniscus have with regard to surgical management of meniscal tears?

What is the gold-standard meniscus repair technique and what are the indications for repair rather than resection of meniscal tears?

What pathology does this arthroscopic view of the medial compartment of the knee show?

It demonstrates a horizontal cleavage tear of the MM that is being probed. The articular surfaces are well preserved.

How can meniscal tears be described?

Tears can be described by:

1. Location, i.e. relevance to blood supply (see question 4)
   - Red zone (outer third)
   - Red–white zone (middle third)
   - White zone (inner third)
2. Morphological pattern of tear
   - Vertical/longitudinal
   - Bucket handle (a large vertical tear that may displace into the notch)
   - Parrot beak (oblique)
   - Radial
   - Horizontal cleavage (common in degenerate tears and may be associated with meniscal cysts)

What is the main function of the meniscus and what clinical relevance does this have with regard to meniscectomy?

The main function of the meniscus is load transmission, which results in reduction of the peak contact stresses in the tibiofemoral compartment. The MM transmits approximately 50% and the lateral meniscus approximately 70% of applied loads in their respective compartments. Meniscectomy results in loss of the distribution of hoop stresses with subsequent point loading on a relatively small surface area, which ultimately results in articular cartilage degeneration. Owing to the higher percentage of applied loads carried by the lateral meniscus, and the fact that the femoral and tibial surfaces on the lateral compartment are both convex, lateral meniscectomy is associated with a higher risk of developing articular degenerative changes (in comparison with medial meniscectomy).

What are the other functions of the meniscus?

- Improvement of articular conformity
- Stability (MM is a secondary AP stabilizer)
- Joint lubrication by distribution of synovial fluid
- Prevention of impingement of the joint capsule during knee motion

What clinical relevance does the blood supply of the meniscus have with regard to surgical management of meniscal tears?

The blood supply of the medial and lateral meniscus is derived from the medial and lateral genicular arteries, respectively (via the perimeniscal capillary plexus). The outer/peripheral portion has a richer blood supply compared with the inner portion (which is practically avascular). The vascular zones are divided into thirds of the cross-section and are named accordingly:

- Red zone (outer third)
- Red–white zone (middle third)
- White zone (inner third)

Thus, I would aim to repair peripheral (outer-third) tears since they have the highest healing potential, whereas inner-third tears have almost no healing potential so I would often resect these.

What is the gold-standard meniscus repair technique, and what are the indications for repair rather than resection of meniscal tears?

The gold-standard repair technique is an inside-out technique using vertical mattress sutures. (One must be aware of damage to neurovascular structures—laterally the common peroneal nerve is at risk, whereas medially it is the saphenous nerve and great saphenous vein.)

Indications for repair can be divided into:

- Location (i.e. relation to blood supply): I would repair peripheral tears in the red zone whenever possible
- Tear morphology: I would aim to repair vertical or longitudinal tears that are greater than 1 cm
- Tissue quality: I would resect chronic degenerate tears back to a stable rim

NB the best results for repair have been achieved in acute red zone tears that are repaired at the same time as ACL reconstruction in a young patient.

Chapter 10   Hip

Viva 81

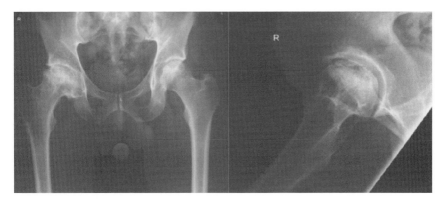

Figure 10.1 A radiograph of a pelvis.

Reproduced from C. Bulstrode et al., *Oxford Textbook of Trauma and Orthopaedics* second edition, 2011, figure 7.16.1, p. 619, with permission from Oxford University Press.

What is the aetiology and what risk factors are associated with avascular necrosis of the femoral head? What other areas are commonly affected?

Can you describe any classification systems for this condition? What stage is shown in the radiographs above?

How would you manage a patient presenting with this condition? What treatment options are available?

What is the aetiology and what risk factors are associated with avascular necrosis of the femoral head? What other areas are commonly affected?

Osteonecrosis (avascular necrosis/aseptic necrosis) occurs within bone following loss of osseous blood supply. All cells within the area of affected bone die away; initially the organic and inorganic matrix are unaffected. It commonly affects patients in the third, fourth, or fifth decade of life. The aetiology of osteonecrosis is still not fully understood and is likely to be multifactorial. Factors thought to contribute to the disruption of the microcirculation include:

- Trauma—leading to macro- and microvascular interruption
- Intravascular coagulation and thrombotic occlusion of microcirculation
- Extravascular compression ('compartment syndrome' within bone) secondary to raised intraosseous pressures

Conditions associated with osteonecrosis include:

- Trauma
- High alcohol intake
- Corticosteroid usage
- Haemoglobinopathy (sickle)
- Hypercoagulation disorders
- Caisson disease (dysbaric osteonecrosis)
- Systemic lupus erythematosus (SLE)
- Ionizing radiation
- Gaucher's disease
- Idiopathic (40%)

Other areas most commonly affected are: the medial femoral condyle, humeral head, talus, lunate (Kienböck's disease), capitellum (Panner's disease), tarsal navicular (Köhler's disease), and metatarsal head (Freiberg's disease).

Can you describe any classification systems for this condition? What stage is shown in the radiographs above?

There are many classification systems described for osteonecrosis of the hip. The Ficat and Arlet (1980) system describes worsening X-ray appearances in four stages and is one of the simplest to use.

The radiographs show Ficat and Arlet stage 3 changes. There is distortion and collapse of the femoral head. The arrow on the lateral view illustrates the 'crescent sign' associated with subchondral collapse.

How would you manage a patient presenting with this condition? What treatment options are available?

Treatment of early osteonecrosis of the femoral head aims to relieve pain and preserve the congruency of the hip joint. In the later stages of the disease arthroplasty procedures are usually required. Investigations used to help stage the disease include: plain radiography, bone scans, and magnetic resonance imaging (MRI).

Early stages (pre-collapse) treatment may include:

- Observation and analgesia
- Treatment of any underlying medical conditions

- Protected weight bearing (little evidence)
- Core decompression +/− bone grafting or vascularized grafts

Later stages (post-collapse):

- Realignment osteotomy
- Arthrodesis
- Replacement arthroplasty (conventional total hip arthroplasty or resurfacing)

Viva 82

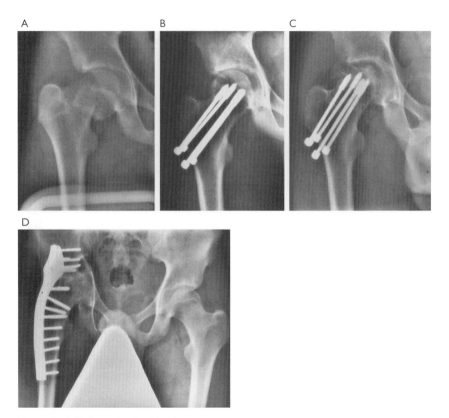

Figure 10.2 Radiographs of a right hip.
Courtesy of Dr S.L. Weinstein.

What considerations need to be taken into account prior to performing a hip arthrodesis?

In what position would you choose to arthrodese a hip?

What are the indications and pre-operative investigations you would perform prior to 'taking down' an arthrodesed hip and converting to a total hip arthroplasty?

What considerations need to be taken into account prior to performing a hip arthrodesis?

Hip arthrodesis, although uncommonly performed, is a useful procedure in the management of younger patients with end-stage unilateral hip disease who have contraindications for replacement or joint-preserving operations. Hip arthrodesis can provide long-term pain relief and stability to the joint. If performed correctly it can allow the patient to have a surprising amount of mobility and return to an active lifestyle.

Requirements for hip arthrodesis:

- Normal contralateral hip
- Normal ipsilateral knee
- Normal lumbar spine
- No significant cardiovascular pathology

Long-term follow-up studies following hip arthrodesis have shown that the majority of patients develop lower back pain and ipsilateral knee pain 20 years or more after the fusion [Callaghan, J.J., Brand, R.A., and Pedersen, D.R. (1985) Hip arthrodesis. A long-term follow-up. *J Bone Joint Surg Am* 67, 1328–35]. The altered gait produced following arthrodesis has been shown to increase oxygen consumption by 32%—this may cause problems in patients with significant cardiovascular pathology.

In what position would you choose to arthrodese a hip?

The recommended position for hip arthrodesis is 20–25° of flexion, slight external rotation, and slight adduction. Internal rotation and abduction should be avoided. Care should be taken at the time of surgery to try and preserve the abductor muscle mass in case a total hip arthroplasty is performed in the future.

What are the indications and pre-operative investigations you would perform prior to 'taking down' an arthrodesed hip and converting to a total hip arthroplasty?

The indications to convert an arthrodesis to a total hip arthroplasty include:

- Increasing low back pain (LBP)/radicular pain
- Contralateral hip disease
- Increasing ipsilateral knee pain
- Painful pseudoarthrosis of the hip

Conversion of an arthrodesed hip to a total hip arthroplasty is a technically demanding procedure. Loss of the normal anatomical landmarks and supporting structures can lead to difficulty in restoring 'normal' joint stability and mechanics. The patient must be fully assessed prior to surgery.

Investigations may include:

- Radiographs to assess bone stock and determine what metalwork (if any) needs to be removed
- Neurophysiology and/or MRI assessment of the abductor muscle mass
- The potential for reactivation of dormant infection must be considered and appropriate biopsies taken pre- or intra-operatively.

Viva 83

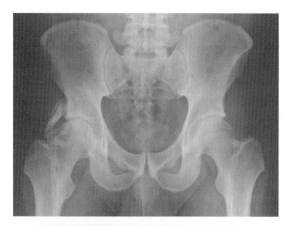

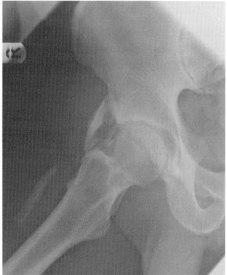

Figure 10.3 AP and lateral radiographs of a right hip.

What do you understand by the term heterotopic ossification (HO)?

How can this affect patients clinically following hip arthroplasty surgery?

Are you aware of any risk factors for developing HO and what measures can you take to try and prevent this condition developing?

How do you manage established HO?

What do you understand by the term heterotopic ossification (HO)?

HO is the process by which mature lamellar bone forms outside the skeleton—usually in soft tissue. Causes include: trauma, neurological injury, severe burns, and genetic conditions (fibrodysplasia ossificans progressiva).

How can this affect patients clinically following hip arthroplasty surgery?

HO following hip arthroplasty surgery is usually asymptomatic and noted as an incidental finding on post-operative radiographs. If the condition becomes severe it can present with restricted and/or painful movement.

HO is most commonly classified using the Brooker system:

Grade 1: Islands of bone lay within the soft tissue around the hip
Grade 2: Boney spurs protrude from either the femur or pelvis, with a gap of more than 1 cm between the spurs
Grade 3: Gaps between the bone spurs are < 1 cm
Grade 4: Apparent ankylosis of the joint

Are you aware of any risk factors for developing HO and what measures can you take to try and prevent this condition developing?

Risk factors for developing HO around the hip include:

- Male gender
- History of HO in either hip
- Ankylosing spondylitis
- Paget's disease
- Pre-existing hip arthrodesis
- Old age
- Diffuse idiopathic skeletal hyperostosis
- Post-traumatic arthritis

Patients at high risk of developing HO or those undergoing surgery to remove HO are often given prophylactic treatment in the peri-operative period. The two main treatments available are non-steroidal anti-inflammatory drugs (NSAIDs) and radiation therapy. Indomethacin is typically given at a dose of 25 mg three times a day for 5–6 weeks after surgery. Low-dose radiation therapy may also be given, typically 7–8 Gy shortly before surgery or up to 72 h post-operatively.

How do you manage established HO?

Management of established HO may be conservative or operative. Initial treatment usually involves physical therapy to try and improve mobility and range of movement in the affected joint. There is no evidence for the use of NSAIDs or radiotherapy in the management of established disease. Surgical excision may be performed if conservative measures fail. Most centres would advocate waiting until maturation of ossification prior to performing the excision (often > 6 months). Particular care should be taken at the time of surgery to clearly identify the neurovascular structures as they may be involved in the ossified tissue.

Viva 84

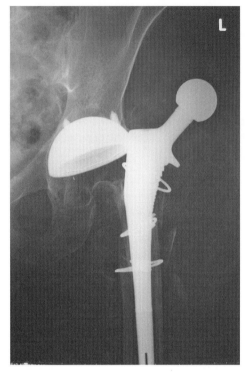

Figure 10.4 A radiograph of a left hip.

Reproduced from C. Bulstrode et al., *Oxford Textbook of Trauma and Orthopaedics* second edition, 2011, figure 7.10.4, p. 586, with permission from Oxford University Press.

What dislocation rate do you quote when consenting a patient for a total hip replacement?

What causes a hip to dislocate?

What measures can you take to prevent re-dislocation?

What dislocation rate do you quote when consenting a patient for a total hip replacement?

Dislocation following hip arthroplasty is one of the most common complications. Large studies have shown the incidence of dislocation following primary hip arthroplasty to be 3–5% over the life of the implant. The dislocation rate more than triples after revision hip surgery. The majority of dislocations occur in the first month (approximately 1%) and year (approximately 2%). Over 50% of hips re-dislocate after initial closed reduction. Dislocation produces significant cost implications—both in terms of patient morbidity and the financial costs of treatment. It has been estimated that the cost of re-operation for a primary dislocation is 150% that of the original surgery.

What causes a hip to dislocate?

Causes of dislocation are multifactorial and can be divided broadly into surgical factors, patient factors, and implant design factors.

- Surgical factors:
  - Component malposition (most common)
  - Soft-tissue imbalance or failure of reattachment
  - Soft-tissue impingement (osteophytes/capsule)
  - Retained debris (cement) in acetabular component
- Patient factors:
  - Previous hip surgery or arthroplasty
  - Female gender (relative risk 2.1)
  - Acute fracture of proximal femur (relative risk 1.8)
  - Inflammatory arthropathy
  - Generalized soft-tissue laxity
  - Patient non-compliance (dementia, learning difficulties, drug/alcohol addiction)
- Implant design factors:
  - Small head/neck ratios—leading to greater impingement risk
  - Small head size (relative risk 1.7 with size 22 mm heads compared with 32 mm)
  - Loosening of components leading to rotation and malalignment
  - Wear of acetabular component leading to head subluxation

What measures can you take to prevent re-dislocation?

Prevention of re-dislocation can be attempted using conservative or operative methods. Assessment of joint stability should be made at the time of reduction. If the hip dislocates in the patient's normal functional range then it is likely that surgical intervention will be required.

Conservative methods

- Patient education/carer advice
- Physiotherapy and occupational therapy input
- Bracing of joint—in an attempt to 'remind the patient' and prevent position of instability

Surgical methods

- Soft-tissue laxity correction:
  - Reattachment of avulsed soft tissues or trochanter
  - Increasing neck offset using modular components
  - Increasing acetabular lateral offset (lateralized liner)
  - Trochanteric advancement

- Increasing range of motion:
  - Increase head–neck ratio (larger femoral head)
  - Excision of osteophytes or soft tissues
  - Increase excursion distance to dislocation (larger femoral head)
  - Revision of malaligned components
- Increase constraint:
  - Augmentation of acetabular liners
  - Constrained or captured liners

Viva 85

This 40-year-old woman presents with increasing pain in her left hip that is associated with severe restriction of function and an apparent leg-length discrepancy.

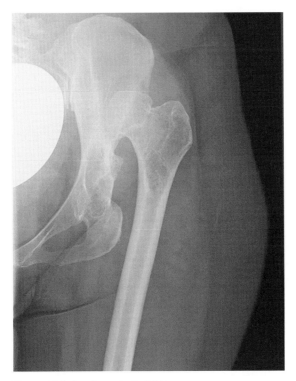

Figure 10.5 A radiograph of a left hip.

What is your diagnosis and how would you classify this condition?

What radiological parameters are used to assess the severity of this condition?

What are the important anatomical considerations when considering a total hip arthroplasty? What other imaging modality is of value pre-operatively?

What are the potential problems that you could encounter and must anticipate when considering a total hip arthroplasty?

What are the possible complications?

What is your diagnosis and how would you classify this condition?

There is a high dislocation of the left hip and secondary osteoarthritis of the joint. The underlying diagnosis is developmental dysplasia of the hip joint. It can be described based on the Crowe Classification system:

- Crowe 1: < 50% subluxation
- Crowe 2: 50–75% subluxation
- Crowe 3: 75–100% subluxation
- Crowe 4: >100% subluxation

An alternative classification system is that proposed by Hartofilakidis. This consists of three groups: 'dysplasia', 'low dislocation', and 'high dislocation'. I would classify this case as a Crowe 4 or 'high dislocation'.

What radiological parameters are used to assess the severity of this condition?

- Lateral centre-edge angle:
  - Normal: > 25°
  - Borderline: between 20 and 25°
  - Dysplastic: < 20°
- Tönnis (sourcil) angle:
  - Normal: < 10°
  - Abnormal: > 10°

What are the important anatomical considerations when planning a total hip arthroplasty? What other imaging modality is of value pre-operatively?

I would obtain a pre-operative computerized tomography (CT) scan to help me assess the morphology and orientation of the acetabulum and femoral head/neck. This CT scan would also demonstrate the degree of acetabular bone deficiency.

What are the potential problems that you could encounter and must anticipate when considering a total hip arthroplasty?

The main issue is restoration of the normal hip centre, i.e. whether to place the acetabular component in an anatomic (inferior) or a non-anatomic (superior/high hip centre) position. Reconstruction with a high hip centre is technically easier and utilizes the host's own iliac bone, thus negating the need for bone grafting. However, the disadvantages include: a persistent limp, higher dislocation rate, and increased rates of component loosening (higher shear forces). I therefore prefer to place the acetabular component at the site of the true acetabulum. The main difficulties I may encounter when attempting this are anterolateral bone deficiency, identification of the true acetabulum, and risk of over-reaming/medialization. It may therefore be necessary to reconstruct the acetabulum using femoral head allograft (bone block and screws) or porous metal augments in order to obtain adequate head coverage.

On the femoral side, restoring the normal hip centre often requires a subtrochanteric femoral shortening osteotomy to prevent significant leg lengthening and the subsequent risk of a traction injury to the sciatic nerve. I would also consider using intra-operative nerve monitoring in such situations.

What are the possible complications?

In addition to the general risks of a total hip replacement, the risks specific to such cases include: nerve injury (sciatic and femoral), vascular injury (a consequence of the approach to the dysplastic acetabulum), and non-union of the femoral osteotomy.

Chapter 11   Spine

Viva 86

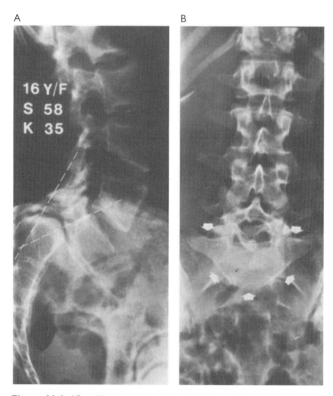

A   B

Figure 11.1 AP and lateral radiographs of a lumbar spine.

What do you understand by the term 'isthmic spondylolisthesis'?

What are the other recognized causes of spondylolisthesis?

How would you grade spondylolisthesis and what radiographic indices maybe used to predict progression?

How do degenerative listheses differ from spondylolysis when considering neural involvement?

What do you understand by the term 'isthmic spondylolisthesis'?

Spondylolisthesis is an anterior sagittal plane translation of a vertebra upon the adjacent caudal level. Isthmic spondylolistheses are secondary to defects in the pars interarticularis at that level. It is most commonly seen at the lumbosacral junction with defects in L5. The spondylolysis is considered to be secondary to mechanical factors leading to a stress fracture of the pars often in sports delivering impact forces to the hyperlordosed lumbar spine in a genetically predisposed population.

What are the other recognized causes of spondylolisthesis?

The other forms of spondylolisthesis as described by Wiltse and Newman are Type I dysplastic, Type II isthmic, Type III degenerative, Type IV traumatic, Type V pathologic, and Type VI iatrogenic.

How would you grade spondylolisthesis and what radiographic indices may be used to predict progression?

Meyerding graded lateral radiographs I–IV sequentially for each 25% slippage with spondyloptosis being a complete slip without endplate to endplate contact. Standing lateral radiographs can be assessed for pelvic incidence, sacral slope, pelvic tilt, and lumbosacral angle, which have all been quoted as predictors of progression. Effectively all these parameters look at lumbosacral shear.

How do degenerative listheses differ from spondylolysis when considering neural involvement?

The striking difference is when the posterior elements are considered. In isthmic spondylolisthesis, the lamina of the affected level remains posteriorly placed and thus central and lateral recess stenosis are seen much less commonly than foraminal stenosis. In these cases a combination of degenerate disc, residual (cephalad pars interarticularis), and reduced foraminal height below the displace pedicle results in radiculopathy. This contrasts with degenerative slips where all three forms of neural encroachment can be seen resulting in a broader spectrum of symptoms.

Viva 87

A 67-year-old male falls onto his face and presents with an abnormal neurological examination and neck pain.

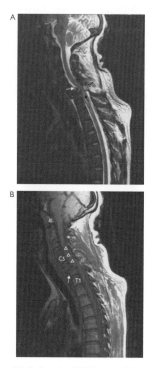

Figure 11.2 A sagittal MRI scan of the neck.

Reproduced from Hadi Manji, Adrian Wills, Neil Kitchen, Neil Dorward, Sean Connelly, and Amrish Mehta, *Oxford Handbook of Neurology*, 2006, figure 5.35, p. 399, with permission from Oxford University Press.

What do you see?

What is the most likely pattern of incomplete cord injury?

What are the clinical features of this injury and how would you manage the patient?

How do the clinical features of Brown–Sequard syndrome differ?

Are you aware of a grading system for cord injury?

How do you grade motor strength and test upper extremity myotomes?

What is spinal shock?

What do you see?

This is a T2-weighted sagittal magnetic resonance imaging (MRI) scan demonstrating cervical spine stenosis at the C5/6 level secondary to a disc prolapse and ligamentum hypertrophy. There is high signal within the cord in keeping with oedema at the C5/6 level.

What is the most likely pattern of incomplete cord injury?

Central cord syndrome.

What are the clinical features of this injury and how would you manage the patient?

There will be predominantly motor rather than sensory deficit affecting the upper extremity more than the lower extremity. It is not unusual to see marked early neurological recovery in such cases, and where no spinal instability exists non-operative management is the standard of care. However, in patients who plateau with a functional disability in conjunction with image-proven cord impingement, surgical decompression and stabilization should be considered.

How do the clinical features of Brown–Sequard syndrome differ?

Brown–Sequard is cord hemisection characterized by: ipsilateral motor weakness, loss of proprioception and tactile discrimination, contralateral pain, and temperature and light touch deficit. There is anecdotal evidence to suggest somewhat better functional prognosis than central cord and anterior cord syndromes.

Are you aware of a grading system for cord injury?

The American Spinal Injury Association (ASIA) scale (AIS):

A = Complete. No sensory or motor function is preserved in the sacral segments S4–5

B = Sensory incomplete. Sensory but not motor function is preserved below the neurological level and includes the sacral segments S4–5 (light touch or pin prick at S4–5 or deep anal pressure) AND no motor function is preserved more than three levels below the motor level on either side of the body

C = Motor incomplete. Motor function is preserved at the most caudal sacral segments for voluntary anal contraction (VAC) OR the patient meets the criteria for sensory incomplete status (sensory function preserved at the most caudal sacral segments S4–5 by light touch [LT], pin prick [PP], or deep anal pressure [DAP]), and has some sparing of motor function more than three levels below the ipsilateral motor level on either side of the body. (This includes key or non-key muscle functions to determine motor incomplete status.) For AIS C—less than half of key muscle functions below the single neurological level of injury (NLI) have a muscle grade ≥ 3

D = Motor incomplete. Motor incomplete status as defined above, with at least half (half or more) of key muscle functions below the single NLI having a muscle grade ≥ 3

E = Normal. If sensation and motor function as tested with the International Standards for Neurological Classification of Spinal Cord Injury (ISNCSCI) are graded as normal in all segments, and the patient had prior deficits, then the AIS grade is E. Someone without an initial spinal cord injury (SCI) does not receive an AIS grade

Using ND: to document the sensory, motor, and NLI levels, the AIS grade, and/or the zone of partial preservation (ZPP) when they are unable to be determined based on the examination results.

How do you grade motor strength and test upper extremity myotomes?

As described on the ISNCSCI worksheet, muscle functions are graded as follows (0–5):

    0 = Total paralysis
    1 = Palpable/visible contraction
    2 = Active, gravity eliminated
    3 = Active against gravity
    4 = Active against some resistance
    5 = Normal power for the individual

To test upper extremity myotomes: C5, elbow flexion; C6, wrist extension; C7, elbow extension; C8, long finger flexors; T1, finger abduction.

© 2020 American Spinal Injury Association. Reprinted with permission.

What is spinal shock?

A transient physiological state, characterized by loss of reflexes and sensorimotor function below the injury level. End of spinal shock is demonstrated by the return of the bulbo-cavernosus reflex (polysynaptic versus monosynaptic).

Viva 88

A 25-year-old man injures his neck after diving into the shallow end of a swimming pool.

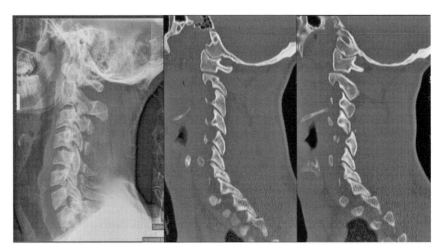

Figure 11.3 A lateral radiograph of the neck, with sagittal CT slices.

What do the images show?

How would you manage the patient?

How would you reduce injury?

What approach would you use to perform a cervical discectomy?

What do the images show?

The lateral cervical spine radiograph shows a subluxation of C4 on C5 of approximately 25%. The subsequent sagittal computerized tomography (CT) reconstructions taken through the facet joints show a unilateral facet joint dislocation at C4/5.

How would you manage the patient?

I would manage the patient according to Advanced Trauma Life Support (ATLS) protocols and immobilize the cervical spine. I would assess and document the neurological status. The immediate goal is to reduce the dislocation and prevent the patient developing a neurological deficit. This can be achieved through a closed or open technique. If the patient has no neurological deficit I would look to obtain an MRI scan to establish if there is an associated disc prolapse. This could potentially be displaced into the cord as the facet is reduced. A disc prolapse would require a discectomy to be performed prior to the reduction. In the case of the patient who has an established deficit or evolving neurology, the priority is to reduce the dislocation as soon as possible with an open or closed technique depending on the skill set of the surgeon. Once the dislocation has been reduced the C4/5 segment would need to be fused surgically.

How would you reduce injury?

A closed reduction can be performed by applying Gardener Wells tongs to the skull in line with the auditory meatus. The patient is kept conscious with sedation so that their neurology can be monitored. Weights are applied gradually using fluoroscopy to monitor the reduction. As a guide 2.5 kg for the head and 0.5 kg for each vertebra is applied to achieve reduction. In those cases where reduction cannot be achieved by traction alone open reduction can be achieved via a posterior approach to the dislocated facet. The facet can be reduced directly or by using a high-speed burr to remove part of the superior facet of C5 allowing the inferior C4 facet to reduce.

What approach would you use to perform a cervical discectomy?

I would perform a Smith–Robinson approach. The patient is placed in a supine position with the shoulders taped down to allow fluoroscopic visualization of the spine. A transverse incision is made to one side of the neck over the affected level between the midline and the anterior border of the sternocleidomastoid. The platysma is divided and a surgical plane is identified between the oesophagus medially and the carotid sheath laterally using blunt dissection. The plane is developed to the prevertebral fascia, which is then divided to expose the anterior longitudinal ligament and the longus coli muscles. The longus coli muscles are elevated from the front of the spine subperiostealy to allow retractor placement and protect the sympathetic chain. The disc level is then confirmed using fluoroscopy.

Viva 89

A 74-year-old gentleman with a colostomy presents with acute onset of left-leg weakness.

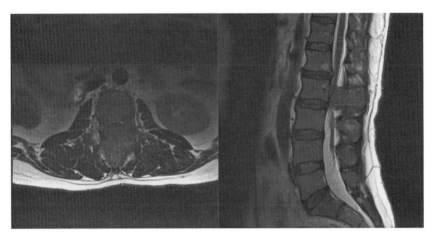

Figure 11.4 MRI sagittal and axial slices of the lumbar spine.

What is this investigation and what does it demonstrate?

How would you manage this patient?

What role does surgery have in these patients?

What is this investigation and what does it demonstrate?

These are T2-weighted sagittal and axial MRI scans of the lumbar spine [the cerebrospinal fluid (CSF) shows up as high signal]. They show a compressive lesion originating from the posterior elements of the lumbar spine. This could be caused by a metastatic lesion, infection, or a primary bone tumour. My main differential would be a metastatic lesion causing cord compression.

How would you manage this patient?

I would investigate for a primary tumour by requesting a CT of the chest, abdomen, and pelvis, as well as bloods for prostate specific antigen and myeloma screen. I would also image the rest of the spine to look for further metastatic deposits. A bone biopsy would provide the best information regarding the source of the lesion. I would manage this patient in accordance with the national guidelines on metastatic cord compression. I would take an multidisciplinary team approach and liaise with the designated lead for metastatic cord compression in my institution. After a full assessment including a detailed neurological examination I would start intravenous (IV) steroids (16 mg dexamethasone) and obtain blood biochemistry to ensure the patient does not have hypercalcaemia. In this case I would consider surgical decompression with posterior pedicle screw stabilization in order to preserve neurological function, control local spread, and maintain spinal stability.

What role does surgery have in these patients?

The goals of surgery in the metastatic spine include: pain control, stabilization, control of local spread, and maintaining continence and mobility. Patchell et al. have demonstrated that surgery has benefits over radiotherapy in treating metastatic spinal disease. Their randomized controlled trial in 2005 was stopped early as patients undergoing surgery vs radiotherapy were found to walk and maintain continence for longer up until their death. A discussion with their oncologist should be sought to establish their life expectancy. The patient's prognosis would need to be greater than 3 months before considering surgery. Patients with intractable pain, lytic lesions, evidence of collapse or deformity, or lesions in junctional regions may potentially benefit from spinal surgery.

Patients with metastatic renal and thyroid disease should have the metastatic area embolized prior to surgery to reduce intra-operative bleeding.

Viva 90

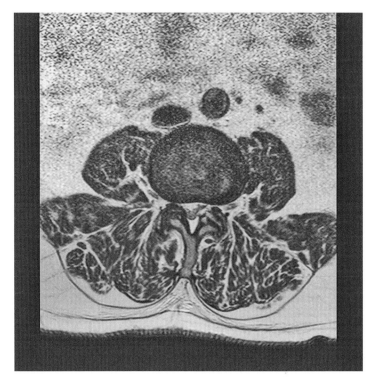

Figure 11.5 An axial MRI scan of the lumbar spine.

Describe the picture above and name the condition that is demonstrated.

What is the common clinical presentation for this condition?

Is there an anatomical classification for the condition?

What would be your indications for surgery in this condition?

When would you perform a fusion in this condition?

Describe the picture above and name the condition that is demonstrated

This is an axial MRI scan (T2-weighted) that shows hypertrophy of the facet joints, hypertrophy of the ligamentum flavum, and a broad-based protrusion of the intervertebral disc resulting in severe stenosis. The condition is spinal stenosis.

What is the common clinical presentation for this condition?

The patient is usually middle aged or older and typically describes gradual onset of low back, buttock, thigh, and calf pain. They may also have numbness, pins and needles, or weakness. The symptoms are exacerbated by walking or even standing. Sitting down or adopting a flexed position of the spine, e.g. pushing a shopping trolley, often relieves the pain.

Is there an anatomical classification for the condition?

Degenerate spinal stenosis can be divided into:

Zone 1 or subarticular stenosis
Zone 2 or foraminal or pedicular stenosis
Zone 3 or extraforaminal or exit stenosis

What would be your indications for surgery in this condition?

Persistent significant pain despite adequate conservative treatment, including physiotherapy and analgesia. The patient should be fit enough for general anaesthesia and understand the risk of complications.

When would you perform a fusion in this condition?

The standard operation is decompression. Fusion should be considered in addition when:

- There is a significant spondylolisthesis
- There is progressive scoliosis or kyphosis
- There is removal of 50% or more of the facet joints
- There is fracture of the pars interarticularis
- There is radical excision of the associated disc causing possible anterior destabilization

Viva 91

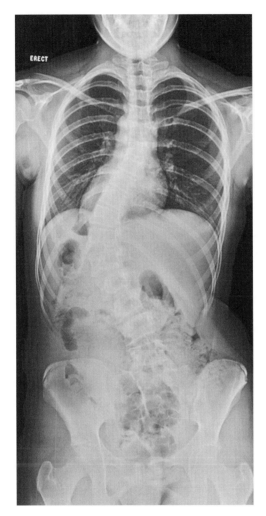

Figure 11.6 Plain X-ray of whole spine.

What is the name of the spinal deformity in the photograph above?

At what age and in which sex does it most commonly present?

What factors affect progression of the deformity?

How is it classified?

What is the name of the spinal deformity in the photograph above?

This is idiopathic scoliosis.

At what age and in which sex does it most commonly present?

It is most common in girls and often presents around adolescence. The thoracic curve is usually right sided. The prevalence is around 3% of the population, although < 10% of curves need treatment.

What factors affect progression of the deformity?

1. The future growth potential of the patient, i.e. the level of skeletal maturity at the time of diagnosis. This is measured by the Risser stage:
   Risser 0 = no ossification of the iliac epiphysis
   Risser 1 = 0–25% ossification
   Risser 2 = 25–50% ossification
   Risser 3 = 50–75% ossification
   Risser 4 = 75–100% ossification
   Risser 5 = fused epiphysis
2. The curve magnitude at the time of diagnosis:
   Curves of < 30° at maturity are unlikely to progress
   Curves of 30–50° at maturity are likely to progress another 10–15°. Curves of > 50° at maturity are likely to progress at around 1°/year
3. Sex: curves in females are more likely to progress
4. Curve type: double curves are more likely to progress

How is it classified?

There are two common classification systems.
   King and Moe describe Types 1–5 depending on the shape of the curve:

Type 1: S-shaped double curve where the lumbar curve is larger or less flexible
Type 2: S-shaped double curve where the thoracic curve is larger or less flexible
Type 3: single thoracic curves
Type 4: long thoracic curves where L4 is tilted into the curve
Type 5: double thoracic curve where T1 is tilted into the thoracic curve

The more complex Lemke classification system describes the curve type (1–6) and adds a modifier (A, B, or C) depending on where the lumbar curve is in relation to the central sacral vertical line, and another modifier (−, N, or +) based on the thoracic sagittal profile.

Viva 92

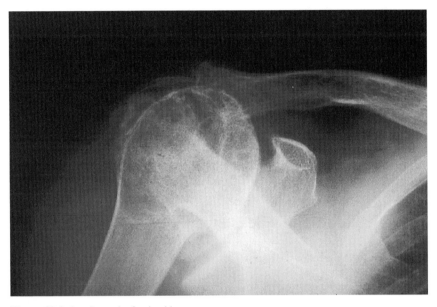

Figure 12.1 A radiograph of a shoulder.

Reproduced from C. Bulstrode et al., *Oxford Textbook of Trauma and Orthopaedics* second edition, 2011, figure 10.3.6, p. 802, with permission from Oxford University Press.

Describe the radiographs. What is your diagnosis?

This is a 70-year-old fit and healthy patient with significant pain and stiffness. She has failed a trial of non-operative treatment. She wants surgery, and a pre-operative scan shows an intact rotator cuff. What will you offer her? Explain how you would consent her.

What surgical approaches are you aware of?

If the patient had a massive cuff tear, what would you do?

Describe the radiographs. What is your diagnosis?

This is an antero-posterior (AP) view of the left shoulder showing a deformed humeral head with loss of joint space and subchondral sclerosis. This is osteoarthritis with a degree of avascular necrosis.

This is a 70-year-old fit and healthy patient with significant pain and stiffness. She has failed a trial of non-operative treatment. She wants surgery, and a pre-operative scan shows an intact rotator cuff. What will you offer her? Explain how you would consent her

In the presence of an intact rotator cuff, I would offer her a shoulder hemiarthroplasty. I would explain to her that the procedure would not restore full movement in her shoulder, although the range of movement is likely to improve. The procedure is very good for pain relief. The procedure would be carried out under general/regional anaesthesia. She is likely to stay in hospital for 2–3 days and will have to wear a sling for approximately 3 weeks and avoid external rotation to protect a repaired tendon (subscapularis). Her mobilization would be monitored by physiotherapists. The risks of the procedure include: infection, injury to nerves and blood vessels, incomplete relief of symptoms, and implant loosening.

What surgical approaches are you aware of?

The procedure can be carried out through a Mackenzie (antero-superior) approach or a delto-pectoral approach.

If the patient had a massive cuff tear, what would you do?

If the patient were to have a massive cuff tear, the outcome following hemiarthroplasty has been reported to be less satisfactory in literature. This patient is unlikely to get any significant relief from non-operative treatments.

I would therefore offer her a reverse total arthroplasty. This has been shown to not only offer good pain relief, but also give the opportunity to improve shoulder function post-operatively. By moving the centre of rotation of the shoulder in an inferior and medial direction, the deltoid muscle can be recruited with good effect to provide an excellent range of motion.

Viva 93

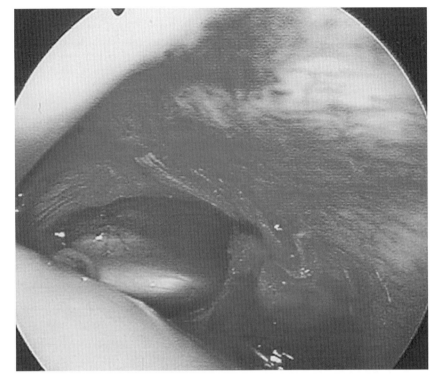

Figure 12.2 An arthroscopic image.
Reproduced from C. Bulstrode et al., *Oxford Textbook of Trauma and Orthopaedics* second edition, 2011, figure 4.5.1, p. 321, with permission from Oxford University Press.

What do you understand by the term 'frozen shoulder'?

What are the classical stages described?

What are the factors associated with this condition?

How would you manage this condition?

Are you aware of any operative procedures for this condition?

What are the typical findings during arthroscopy?

What do you understand by the term 'frozen shoulder'?

Frozen shoulder is the term used to describe the condition in which there is gradual onset of pain in the shoulder followed by stiffness.

What are the classical stages described?

The condition is typically characterized by three stages. Stage 1 is the painful phase, which usually lasts 2–9 months. Patients usually complain of night pain. Stage 2 is the phase of stiffness and usually lasts 4–12 months. All movements are usually affected. Stage 3 is the stage of thawing, which also usually lasts 4–12 months. The stages overlap each other and are not discrete.

What are the factors associated with this condition?

Factors associated with frozen shoulder are diabetes mellitus, trauma, chest disease, rotator cuff tear, hyperlipidaemia, thyroid, and autoimmune disease.

How would you manage this condition?

I will explain the diagnosis and natural history of frozen shoulder. I will offer an intra-articular steroid injection and analgesia, particularly in the painful phase. I will also refer the patient for physiotherapy. If symptoms fail to resolve, I would consider manipulation under anaesthesia or arthroscopic capsular release.

Are you aware of any operative procedures for this condition?

Manipulation under anaesthetic by an experienced shoulder surgeon or arthroscopic capsular release is sometimes necessary for resistant cases.

What are the typical findings during arthroscopy?

The joint feels tight and the rotator interval is narrowed. Marked synovial injection is seen in the rotator interval.

Viva 94

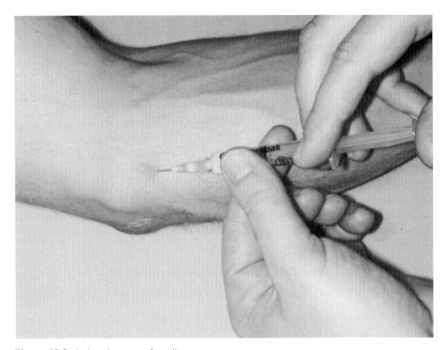

Figure 12.3 A clinical picture of an elbow.

This figure was published in *Orthopedics in Primary Care*, second edition, Andrew J. Carr and William Hamilton. Copyright Elsevier 2004.

What is tennis elbow?

What is the differential diagnosis?

What are the histopathological findings in this condition?

How would you manage this condition?

Describe the surgical procedure you would perform.

What is tennis elbow?

Tennis elbow is a condition characterized by pain in the region of the lateral epicondyle of the elbow; there is sometimes swelling and usually tenderness over the common extensor tendon. Resisted movements of the wrist and finger exteriors are usually painful.

What is the differential diagnosis?

Differential diagnosis includes: cervical spine pathology, radio-capitellar osteoarthropathy, and radial tunnel syndrome/posterior interosseous nerve entrapment.

What are the histopathological findings in this condition?

A histological finding typical of this condition is angiofibroblastic hyperplasia, which represents a degenerative process. The extensor carpi radialis brevis is commonly involved and may have degenerative tears.

How would you manage this condition?

The management is mainly non-operative. I would advise patients on activity modification, analgesia, and use of a brace. I would refer them to physiotherapy. The role of steroids is being disputed. Recent studies have shown no significant beneficial effect with steroids. Surgical release may be necessary, if all non-operative treatments fail.

Describe the surgical procedure you would perform

You should be able to describe the lateral approach to the common extensor origin.

Viva 95

A 19-year-old man competes at rugby at elite level. He dislocated his right shoulder during a match 4 weeks ago. This was his first dislocation. It required reduction in A&E. He has no neurological problems, has regained full range of movement, but his shoulder feels unstable.

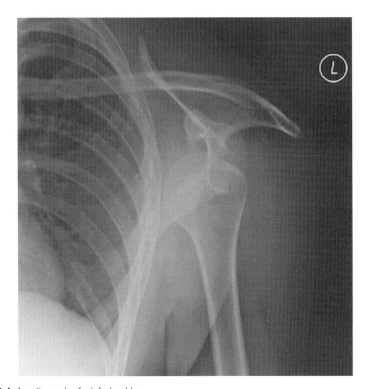

Figure 12.4 A radiograph of a left shoulder.

Reproduced from Philip G. Conaghan, Philip O'Connor, and David A. Isenberg, *Oxford Specialist Handbook: Musculoskeletal Imaging*, figure 4.6, p. 105, 2010, with permission from Oxford University Press.

What type of instability is he most likely to have?

How would you treat him?

What surgical options are available?

Describe the deltopectoral approach.

What type of instability is he most likely to have?

He has traumatic instability; this implies there is a structural defect—traditionally the TUBS (traumatic, unilateral, Bankart lesion, surgery) classification has been used but now the Bailey triangle is used most commonly by shoulder surgeons and this case would be a Bailey type I [a Bailey type II is a traumatic dislocation without a structural defect (the trauma often being less significant) while a Bailey type III is non-traumatic without a structural defect. Placing patients in the correct group helps guide your management.]

How would you treat him?

Surgically, he has had a significant traumatic event with a likely structural defect (the Bankart lesion). He is in a young age group, plays rugby at elite level, and is at high risk of further dislocation. It is perfectly reasonable to proceed directly to surgery. It is reasonable to arrange an MRI arthrogram but some surgeons proceed to surgery based on the history and examination.

What surgical options are available?

A Bankart repair with inferior capsular shift. This can be done both arthroscopically and through an open approach. The key stages are reattachment of the glenoid labrum between the 3 and 6 o'clock position on the right glenoid and the 6 and 9 o'clock on the left glenoid. At the same time an inferior capsular shift is performed, which decreases external rotation. Physiotherapy is very important post-operatively.

Describe the deltopectoral approach

This is a classic approach that you must be able to describe. See Viva 28.

Chapter 13 Tumours

Viva 96

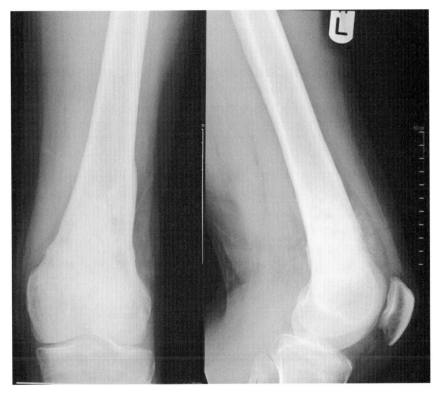

Figure 13.1 Radiographs of a distal femur.

Describe what you see on these radiographs. What do you think is the most likely diagnosis?

How would you investigate this lesion further? What are the principles of performing an open tumour biopsy?

Outline your treatment options once the lesion has been identified and staged. Are you aware of any prognostic indicators?

Describe what you see on these radiographs. What do you think is the most likely diagnosis?

When describing bone lesions remember: age, bone, site, matrix, margin, periosteal reaction, soft tissue mass, and likely diagnoses.

The radiograph shows a lesion arising from the distal femoral metaphysis in a skeletally mature patient. The matrix of the lesion is mostly sclerotic, suggesting osteoblastic (bone-forming) activity; there are also a few small lytic (bone destruction) areas. The margins of the lesion are not clearly defined with a broad zone of transition into the surrounding bone. The cortex of the bone overlying the lesion is poorly defined and has been invaded by the lesion. The periosteum has been elevated anteriorly (Codman's triangle) and there is an associated 'sunburst' spiculation appearance. The lesion appears to have expanded out into the surrounding soft tissues. These features suggest that this is an aggressive, fast-growing, osteoblastic lesion of the distal femur—the most likely diagnosis would be an osteosarcoma.

How would you investigate this lesion further? What are the principles of performing an open tumour biopsy?

Any bone lesion that is suspected of being aggressive or having malignant potential should be thoroughly investigated. Ideally these investigations and the subsequent management should be performed at a specialist tumour centre—early referral is recommended. Investigations are performed to accurately identify and stage the lesion prior to planning definitive treatment. These often include:

1. Local staging (performed prior to biopsy to prevent problems in interpretation):
   Plain radiographs
   Magnetic resonance imaging (MRI)
   Ultrasonography
2. Distant staging:
   Chest X-ray
   Computerized tomography (CT) of chest bone scans
   Positron emission tomography (PET)
3. Lesion identification:
   Blood tests and tumour markers
   Open biopsy
   Tru-cut biopsy
   Fine-needle aspiration

The basic principles of open biopsy should be applied to prevent further seeding and spread of a potentially malignant tumour:

- The biopsy should be performed by the surgeon who will perform any definitive surgery
- No limb exsanguination
- The biopsy tract should easily be removed with the incision for definitive surgery
- Utilize longitudinal extensile approaches, not transverse incisions
- Through compartments (muscle) rather than splitting through tissue planes
- No undermining of skin edges or tissue planes
- Adequate sample size and location—including the periphery of the lesion not just necrotic core tissue
- Immaculate haemostasis
- Drains brought out through or at the edge of the wound for easy tract excision

Outline your treatment options once the lesion has been identified and staged. Are you aware of any prognostic indicators?

Multi-agent chemotherapy in conjunction with surgery is the standard treatment for osteosarcoma. Typically neo-adjuvant chemotherapy is given prior to surgery. The tumour is then re-staged and definitive surgery is performed for local disease control—limb salvage (over 90% of surgery) or amputation options are available depending on the site and stage of the tumour.

Overall 5-year survival rates for osteosarcoma are approximately 60%. Patients with large-volume tumours, metastatic disease, or disease in the axial skeleton tend to fare much worse than those with peripheral and localized disease. Patients in whom a good histopathological response to neo-adjuvant chemotherapy has been achieved (> 95% tumour cell kill or necrosis) have a better prognosis than those whose tumours do not respond as favourably.

Viva 97

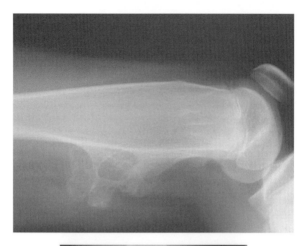

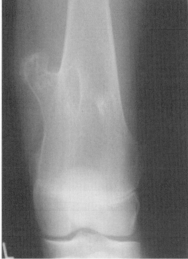

Figure 13.2 Radiographs of a knee.

Describe the abnormalities you see on these radiographs. What is the likely diagnosis?

What is the inheritance pattern and natural history of this disease? What sites are commonly affected?

What clinical problems does it cause?

Describe the abnormalities you see on these radiographs. What is the likely diagnosis?

These antero-posterior (AP) and lateral radiographs show sessile lesions arising from the metaphyseal region of the distal femur. The lesions are well defined and appear to be growing away from the metaphysis. The matrix of the lesions is in continuity with the surrounding normal bone. The cortex of the normal bone appears to be in continuity with the lesions. The caps of the lesions contain specks of calcification. These appearances would be compatible with a slow-growing, benign lesion, most likely osteochondroma.

What is the inheritance pattern and natural history of this disease? What sites are commonly affected?

Hereditary multiple exostoses (HME) is a familial inherited autosomal dominant condition but spontaneous mutation also occurs. Males are more often affected, possibly owing to an incomplete penetrance in females. Three gene mutations have been identified that can lead to HME. HME Type I is caused by a mutation in the gene encoding exostosin-1 (EXT1), which maps to chromosome 8q24. HME Type II is caused by mutation in the gene encoding exostosin-2 (EXT2), on chromosome 11, and HME Type III has been mapped to a locus on chromosome 19 (EXT3). There is some evidence for an additional multiple exostoses locus. The condition has an estimated incidence of 1 in 50,000. Exostoses may be present at birth—over 80% of patients are diagnosed in the first decade of life (median age 3 years). There may be a few or hundreds of lesions present and the number and size tend to increase with growth.

The radiographic distribution of lesions is as follows:

Distal femur 70%
Ribs 40%
Proximal tibia 70%
Distal radius 30%
Proximal humerus 50%
Distal ulna 30%
Scapula 40%

What clinical problems does it cause?

Generally, patients present with a painless mass. The developing exostoses may lead to abnormalities in osseous growth, joint restriction, joint deformities particularly affecting paired bones, and early progression to osteoarthritis.

Lesions that continue to enlarge after the end of puberty are abnormal and should be investigated for potential malignant change (chondrosarcoma). Ultrasonography and MRI are usually the investigations of choice.

Features suggesting malignant change include:

- Increasing pain and swelling (especially after cessation of normal growth)
- Thickening of the cartilage cap (> 2 cm is very concerning)
- Lysis of a proportion of the stalk
- Intramedullary invasion of the underlying bone

Appendix

Diagrams for the FRCS (Tr&Orth)

Questions

There a certain number of diagrams that candidates get asked to draw—here are some that have been asked for in the past.

You should be able to sketch these out quickly. Try to talk and explain as you go so you are gaining points as you draw.

1. Draw and label a growth plate.
2. Draw and label the microscopic structure of muscle.
3. Draw and label the microscopic structure of cortical bone.
4. Draw and label a cross-section of nerve/tendon/meniscus/intravertebral disc.
5. Draw and label a cross-section of the spinal cord.
6. Draw and label a cross-section of articular cartilage.
7. Draw and label a proteoglycan.
8. Draw and label a stress–strain curve for bone/steel/titanium/plastic, etc.
9. Draw and label the brachial plexus/lumbar plexus.
10. Draw and label the flexor/extensor tendon zones of the hand.
11. Draw and label a cross-section of the lower leg/mid-thigh level.
12. Draw and label a screw used in orthopaedics.
13. Draw and label a cross-section through the vertebral column at L4/5.
14. Draw the graph of the tibio-femoral angle from birth to adulthood.
15. Draw and label the zones around a total hip replacement.
16. Draw and label a graph showing how bone mineral density varies with age.
17. Draw out the pathways of calcium homeostasis/vitamin D.
18. Draw and label an inheritance table for an autosomal recessive/autosomal dominant/X-linked condition.
19. Draw and label a Z-plasty.
20. Draw and label a free body diagram of the hip/elbow.
21. Draw and label a skeletal traction system that you know.
22. Draw a bacterium showing where antibiotics act.

Answers

1. **Draw and label a growth plate.**

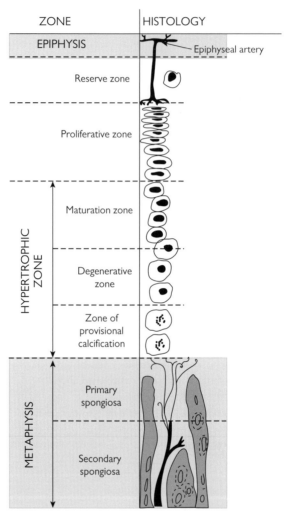

Figure A1 app001

Illustration by Ad Ghande.

2. Draw and label the microscopic structure of muscle.

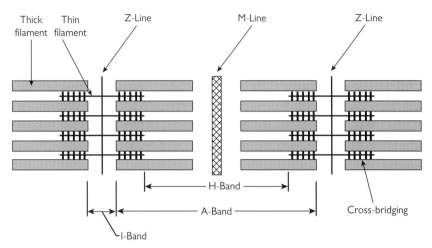

Figure A2 app002

Illustration by Ad Ghande.

3. Draw and label the microscopic structure of cortical bone.

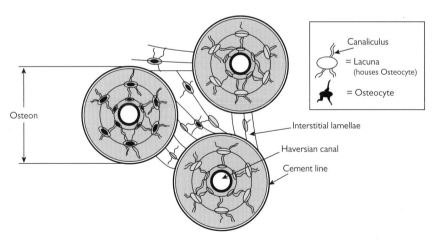

Figure A3 app003

Illustration by Ad Ghande.

4. **Draw and label a cross-section of nerve/tendon/meniscus/ intravertebral disc.**

NERVE

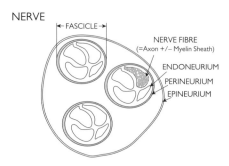

Tendon

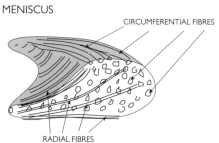

MENISCUS

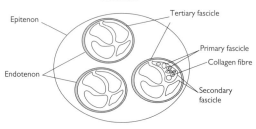

INTERVERTEBRAL DISC

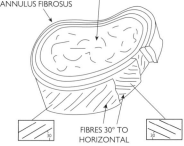

Figure A4 app004

Illustration by Ad Ghande.

5. Draw and label a cross-section of the spinal cord.

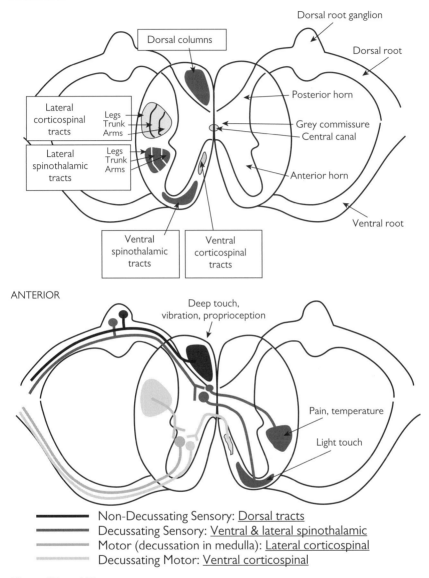

Figure A5 app005

Illustration by Ad Ghande.

6. Draw and label a cross-section of articular cartilage.

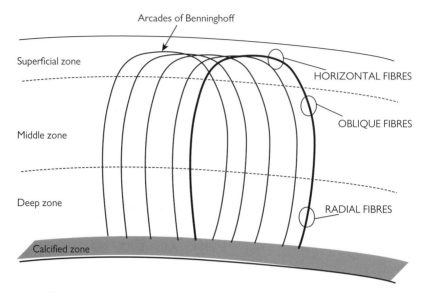

Figure A6 app006

Illustration by Ad Ghande.

7. Draw and label a proteoglycan.

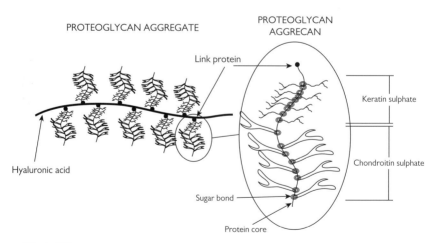

Figure A7 app007

Illustration by Ad Ghande.

8. Draw and label a stress–strain curve for bone/steel/titanium/plastic, etc.

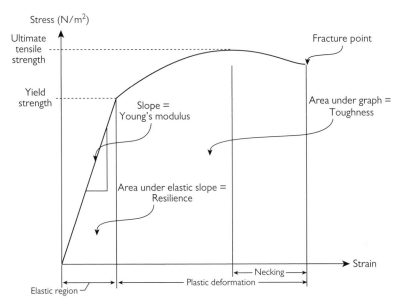

Figure A8 app008

Illustration by Ad Ghande.

9. Draw and label the brachial plexus.

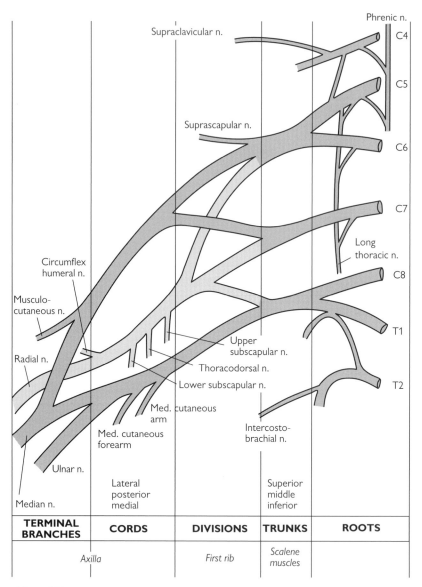

Figure A9 app009

Reproduced from Graeme McLeod, Colin McCartney, and Tony Wildsmith (2012) *Principles and Practice of Regional Anaesthesia* fourth edition, figure 17.1, with permission from Oxford University Press.

10. Draw and label the flexor/extensor tendon zones of the hand.

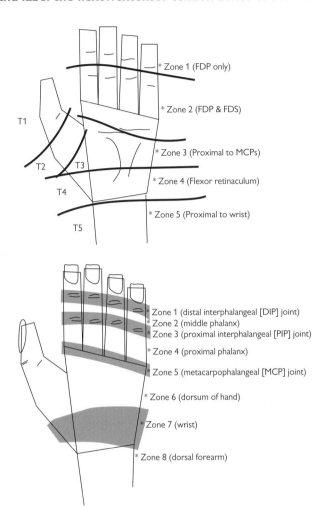

* Zone 1 (FDP only)

* Zone 2 (FDP & FDS)

* Zone 3 (Proximal to MCPs)

* Zone 4 (Flexor retinaculum)

* Zone 5 (Proximal to wrist)

* Zone 1 (distal interphalangeal [DIP] joint)
* Zone 2 (middle phalanx)
* Zone 3 (proximal interphalangeal [PIP] joint)

* Zone 4 (proximal phalanx)

* Zone 5 (metacarpophalangeal [MCP] joint)

* Zone 6 (dorsum of hand)

* Zone 7 (wrist)

* Zone 8 (dorsal forearm)

Figure A10 app010

Illustration by Ad Ghande.

11. Draw and label a cross-section of the lower leg/mid-thigh level.

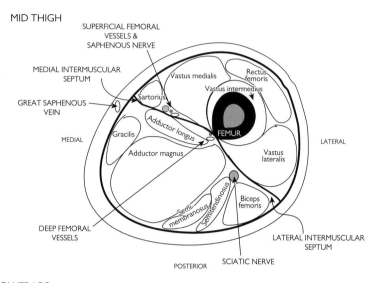

Figure A11 app011

Illustration by Ad Ghande.

12. Draw and label a screw used in orthopaedics.

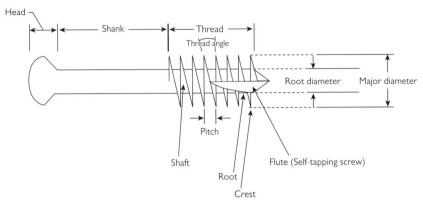

Figure A12 app012

Illustration by Ad Ghande.

13. Draw and label a cross-section through the vertebral column at L4/5.

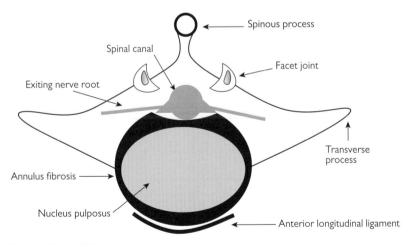

Figure A13 app013

14. Draw the graph of the tibio-femoral angle from birth to adulthood.

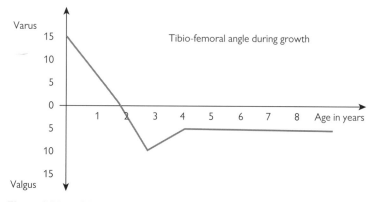

Figure A14 app014

15. Draw and label the zones around a total hip replacement.

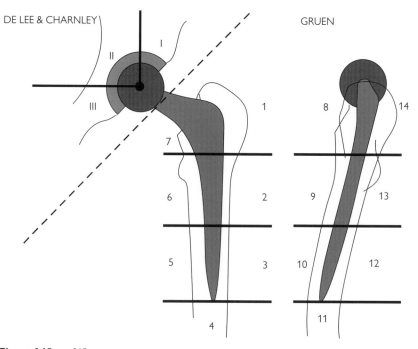

Figure A15 app015

Illustration by Ad Ghande.

16. **Draw and label a graph showing how bone mineral density varies with age.**

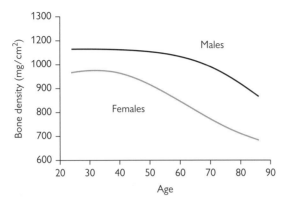

Figure A16 app016

Illustration by Ad Ghande.

17. **Draw out the pathways of calcium homeostasis/vitamin D.**

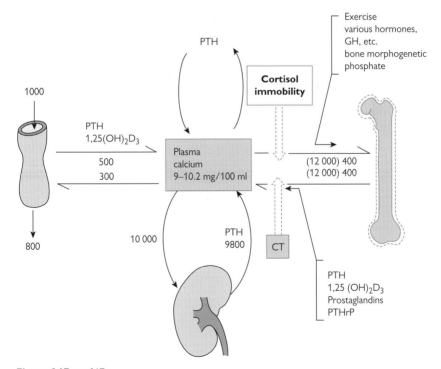

Figure A17 app017

Reproduced from Smith, 1997, *Oxford Textbook of Rheumatology* 2nd edition, Oxford: Oxford University Press, pp. 421–440, with permission.

18. Draw and label an inheritance table for an autosomal recessive/ autosomal dominant/X-linked condition.

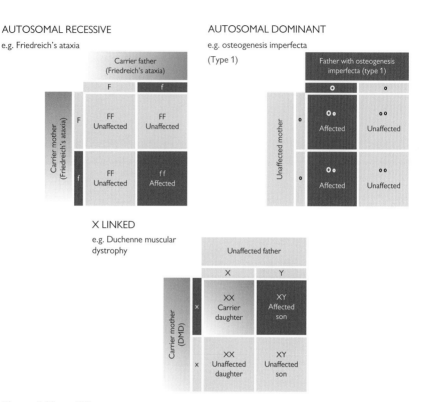

Figure A18 app018

Illustration by Ad Ghande.

19. Draw and label a Z-plasty.

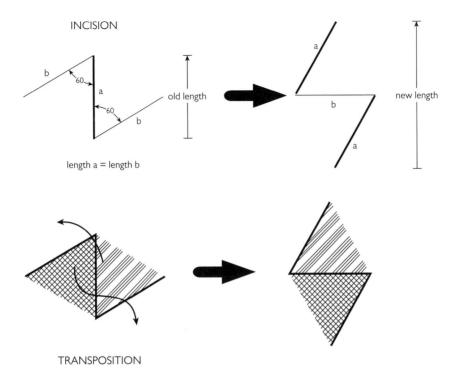

INCISION

length a = length b

old length

new length

TRANSPOSITION

Figure A19 app019

Illustration by Ad Ghande.

20. **Draw and label a free body diagram of the hip/elbow.**

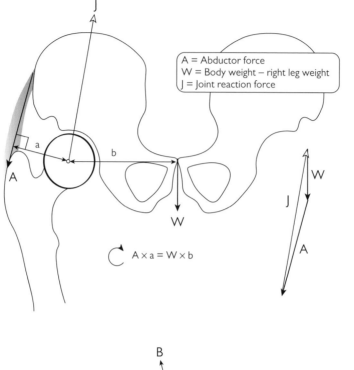

A = Abductor force
W = Body weight – right leg weight
J = Joint reaction force

$A \times a = W \times b$

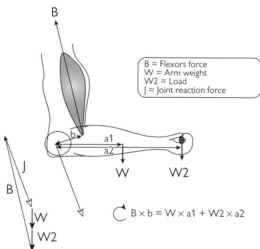

B = Flexors force
W = Arm weight
W2 = Load
J = Joint reaction force

$B \times b = W \times a1 + W2 \times a2$

Figure A20 app020

Illustration by Ad Ghande.

21. **Draw and label a skeletal traction system that you know.**

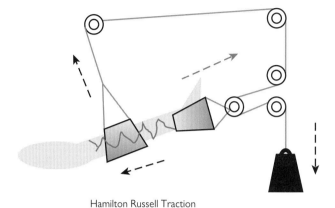

Hamilton Russell Traction

Figure A21 app021

22. **Draw a bacterium showing where antibiotics act.**

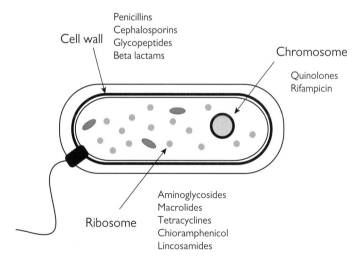

Cell wall

Penicillins
Cephalosporins
Glycopeptides
Beta lactams

Chromosome

Quinolones
Rifampicin

Ribosome

Aminoglycosides
Macrolides
Tetracyclines
Chloramphenicol
Lincosamides

Figure A22 app022

Illustration by Ad Ghande.

List of Abbreviations

AAOS	American Academy of Orthopaedic Surgeons
AC	acromioclavicular
ACF	antecubital fossa
ACL	anterior cruciate ligament
A&E	accident and emergency department
AIS	abbreviated injury scale
AP	antero-posterior
APL	abductor pollicis longus
APTT	activated partial thromboplastin time
ARDS	adult respiratory distress syndrome
ASIA	American Spinal Injury Association
ASIS	anterior superior iliac spine
ATLS	Advanced Trauma Life Support
AVN	avascular necrosis
BAPRAS	British Association of Plastic Reconstructive and Aesthetic Surgeons
BMD	bone mineral density
BMP	bone morphogenic protein
BOA	British Orthopaedic Association
BOAST	British Orthopaedic Association Standards for Trauma and Orthopaedics
BSCOS	British Society for Children's Orthopaedic Surgery
CCP	cyclic citrullinated peptide
CMC	carpo-metacarpal
CMT	Charcot–Marie–Tooth
CPN	Common Peroneal Nerve
CRP	C-reactive protein
CRPS	complex regional pain syndrome
CSF	cerebrospinal fluid
CT	computerized tomography
DAIR	debride and retain
DAP	Deep anal pressure
DCP	dynamic compression plate
DCO	damage control orthopaedics
DDH	developmental dysplasia of the hip
DIP	distal interphalangeal
DISI	dorsal intercalated segment instability
DM	diabetes mellitus

DMAA	distal metatarsal articular angle
DMARD	disease-modifying anti-rheumatic drug
DRU	distal radioulnar
DVT	deep vein thrombosis
ECG	electrocardiogram
ECRB	extensor carpi radialis brevis
ECRL	extensor carpi radialis longus
ECU	extensor carpi ulnaris
ED	extensor digitorum
EDC	extensor digitorum communis
EDM	extensor digiti minimi
EI	extensor indicis
EMG	electromyography
EPB	extensor pollicis brevis
EPL	extensor pollicis longus
ER	external rotation
ESR	erythrocyte sedimentation rate
EUA	examination under anaesthesia
EXT	exostosin
FAST	focused assessment with sonography in trauma
FBC	full blood count
FCR	`flexor carpi radialis
FCU	flexor carpi ulnaris
FDL	flexor digitorum longus
FFD	fixed flexion deformity
FFP	fresh frozen plasma
FH	Family History
GA	general anaesthetic
GABA	gamma-aminobutyric acid
GMFCS	Gross Motor Function Classification System
GT	greater tuberosity
HME	ereditary multiple exostoses
HMSN	hereditary motor sensory neuropathy
HO	heterotopic ossification
HV	hallux valgus
HVIP	hallux valgus interphalangeus
IGHL	inferior glenohumeral ligament
IL	interleukin
IMA	intermetatarsal angle

IML	intermalleolar ligament
INR	international normalized ratio
IPA	interphalangeal angle
ISNCSCI	International Standards for Neurological Classification of Spinal Cord Injury
ISS	injury severity score
IV	intravenous
LBP	low back pain
LCL	lateral collateral ligament
LHB	long head of biceps tendon
LLD	leg-length discrepancy
LMWH	low-molecular-weight heparin
LT	lunotriquetral
MCP1	metacarpophalangeal
MCL	medial collateral ligament
MCR	Midcarpal Radial
MCU	Midcarpal Ulnar
MGHL	middle glenohumeral ligament
MM	medial meniscus
MMA	mono methyl methacrylate
MODS	multiple organ dysfunction syndrome
MRC	Medical Research Council
MRI	magnetic resonance imaging
MT	metatarsal
MTP	metatarsophalangeal
NAI	non-accidental injury
NCS	nerve conduction studies
NICE	National Institute of Health and Clinical Excellence
NLI	Neurological level of injury
NSAID	non-steroidal anti-inflammatory drug
OA	osteoarthritis
ORIF	open reduction and internal fixation
PA	postero-anterior
PCL	posterior cruciate ligament
PDGF	platelet-derived growth factor
PET	positron emission tomography
PF	patello-femoral
PGE2	prostaglandin 2
PIP	proximal interphalangeal
PLC	posterolateral corner

PMMA	pre-polymerized poly methyl methacrylate
PNS	Peripheral Nervous System
POP	plaster of Paris
PP	pin prick
PR	Per Rectum
PROM	patient-reported outcome measure
PS	posterior-stabilized
PTH	parathyroid hormone
PV	Per vaginal
RA	rheumatoid arthritis
RANK	receptor activator of nuclear factor kappa-B
RANKL	receptor activator of nuclear factor kappa-B ligand
RCI	round-headed cannulated interference
RCT	randomized controlled trial
RF	radiofrequency
ROM	range of motion
RSA	Roentgen stereophotogrammetric analysis
RTA	road traffic accident
SC	subcutaneously
SC	supracondylar
SCI	spinal cord injury
SD	standard deviation
SEM	standard error of the mean
SGHL	superior glenohumeral ligament
SI	sacroiliac
SLAC	scaphoid lunate advanced collapse
SLE	systemic lupus erythematosus
SNAC	scaphoid non-union advanced collapse
SUFE	slip of the right upper femoral epiphysis
STT	scapho-trapezio-trapezoidal
TA	tibialis anterior
TFCC	triangular fibrocartilage complex
THR	total hip replacement
TKR	total knee replacement
TNF	tumour necrosis factor
TPT	tibialis posterior tendon
TRAP	tartrate-resistant acid phosphatase
TUBS	traumatic, unilateral, Bankart lesion, surgery
UCL	ulnar collateral ligament

UHMWPE	ultra-high-molecular-weight polyethylene
UKR	unicompartmental knee replacement
UTS	ultimate tensile stress
VAC	voluntary anal contraction
vWF	von Willebrand's factor
WBC	white blood cells
XLPE	cross-linked polyethylene
ZPP	zone of partial preservation

Index

X

Y

Z